20-Minute Yoga
Workouts

BY ALICE CHRISTENSEN:

The American Yoga Association Beginner's Manual

Easy Does It Yoga for Older People

Easy Does It Yoga Trainer's Guide

Meditation

Reflections of Love

The Light of Yoga

The Joy of Celibacy

Conversations with Swami Lakshmanjoo, Volume I
ASPECTS OF KASHMIR SHAIVISM

Conversations with Swami Lakshmanjoo, Volume II
THE YAMAS AND NIYAMAS OF PATANJALI

Basic Yoga (videotape)

Complete Relaxation and Meditation (audiotape)

Conversations with Swami Lakshmanjoo (three-part videotape)

20-Minute Yoga
Workouts

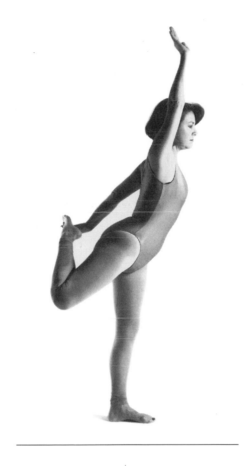

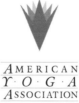

AMERICAN
Y·O·G·A
ASSOCIATION

with Alice Christensen,
Founder, The American Yoga Association

PRODUCED BY THE PHILIP LIEF GROUP, INC.

Ballantine Books • New York

Copyright © 1995 American Yoga Association and
The Philip Lief Group, Inc.

All rights reserved under International and Pan-American Copyright Conventions. Published in the United States by Ballantine Books, a division of Random House, Inc., New York, and simultaneously in Canada by Random House of Canada Limited, Toronto.

Photographs by Evelyn England unless otherwise credited.
The models for this book are Yoga students of the American Yoga Association.

Library of Congress Catalog Card Number: 94-96755

ISBN: 0-345-38845-3

COVER DESIGN BY DAVID STEVENSON
COVER PHOTO BY EVELYN ENGLAND
BOOK DESIGN AND TYPESETTING
BY BETTY BINNS DESIGN

MANUFACTURED IN THE UNITED STATES OF AMERICA
FIRST EDITION: JULY 1995

10 9 8 7 6 5 4 3 2 1

This book is dedicated to Rama,
my great teacher.

CONTENTS

PREFACE

Keats has always been one of my favorite poets. In his short life, he embodied and wrote about an attitude that is very close to the heart of a mystic like me; he called it "negative capability." Negative capability is the ability to be "in uncertainties, Mysteries, doubts, without any irritable reaching after fact and reason." In Yoga, and especially in the philosophical thread of Yoga that I practice and teach, called Kashmir Shaivism, this idea of being able to live happily in uncertainty is the pinnacle of achievement. The experience of Yoga cannot blossom if it is tied to a demand for a certain result. How can we know what the results will be, anyway? One of the beauties of Yoga practice is its infinite possibilities.

To practice Yoga happily and successfully, one must be open to constant change; be ready for anything; be nonjudgmental. As you begin your practice of the 20-minute workout, look forward to Yoga like a surprise package that you will open with no preconceptions of what is inside. I know that change sometimes is frightening because it is unknown. But the unknown can be viewed with two faces: as a possible threat or as a possible opportunity. A person practicing Yoga becomes a strong individual capable of making choices in life.

I have been very fortunate in my life to have known two great masters of Yoga personally. The first, Swami Rama of Haridwar and Kashmir, was a guiding light to me for nearly a decade, and his wisdom and truth continue to support my life and work every day. The second, Swami Lakshmanjoo, was the greatest master of Kashmir Shaivism in a line of teachers stretching back to the great Abhinavagupta and beyond. For nearly 20 years I traveled to Kashmir to study with him each summer. He

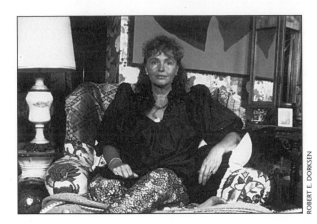

ROBERT E. DORKSEN

introduced me to, and taught me in, the philosophical school of Kashmir Shaivism, a philosophy that views the universe and the whole of life and mind in terms of feeling, and that experiences Yoga as a continuing process of becoming that. I feel privileged to be able to share some of the richness of Yoga technique with you in this book.

The classical tradition of Yoga is teacher to student, one on one. These days, people are more likely to practice in a class or at home alone with a book or videotape than with a personal teacher. I have written this book in a way that allows me to be your teacher through the written word. Consider me your teacher, just as if you were in a daily or weekly class. Write to me if you have questions about what you are doing, or if you have any comments about this book.

I look forward to hearing from you, and I wish you the best of success, enjoyment, and opportunity as you begin your 20-minute Yoga workout.

Alice Christensen
SARASOTA, FLORIDA

ACKNOWLEDGMENTS

*The author wishes to thank the entire staff of the
American Yoga Association for their help in the preparation of this book,
particularly Patricia Hammond, executive editor.*

20-Minute Yoga
Workouts

1

20 MINUTES: THAT'S ALL IT TAKES

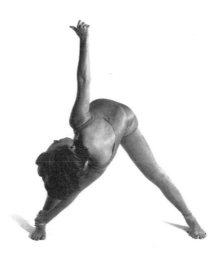

Imagine a workout that psyches you up without tiring you out! That's the 20-minute workout you'll learn in this book. This compact, efficient, energizing, high-power-but-low-impact, all-natural-nothing-artificial program is for you, the person with a lot going on in life. You're involved, you're busy, you're always on your way somewhere. You want an organized workout that gets you going but relaxes that "hyper" feeling —without compromising your many commitments. Perhaps you're also looking for meaning in what you do: a concept of fitness that addresses more than physical culture for its own sake. Maybe you'd like more self-confidence, mental clarity, or concentration.

Why Yoga?

Yoga means union with yourself. Yoga can be a tool for you to use—like the electricity that runs your appliances or the engine that runs your car. It is a powerful connection to yourself, a support system whose many techniques can have many different results, depending on your desires. If you want to relax, Yoga can teach you how to relax every muscle. If you want to stretch, Yoga can limber your joints and stretch your muscles. If you want to learn how to be less angry or tense or reactive, Yoga can teach you how to slow down. If you want to improve your posture, Yoga can elongate and strengthen your back muscles. If you are healing from an addiction, Yoga can help to remove dependence on alcohol or drugs or nicotine. And Yoga can lead you to a new understanding of who you are and show you where the power to be yourself lies. In this book, you will find a variety of applications of Yoga practice that will start you on the way to learning how to use the techniques to best advantage. All it takes is a commitment to 20 minutes a day.

How Can Yoga Do All That in *20 Minutes*?

From the beginning, Yoga was designed for efficiency. Yoga takes no special equipment, and it can be practiced in very small quarters. Those individuals practicing alone in the Himalayan mountains of India thousands of years ago observed what happened to their body, breath, and mind, and how they felt as they experimented with different movements, breath patterns, and methods of concentration. Over time, the techniques of Yoga evolved from this intense personal experience, methodical observation, and creative invention. They were refined and streamlined to provide a quick way to make the body and mind strong, resilient, healthy, and powerful, and to prevent aging.

Hardly anybody these days has the time or inclination to spend many hours a day on Yoga. And because of the work of those early practitioners, it really isn't necessary. "Quality time"—the catchphrase of the 1980s—still applies when it comes to Yoga practice. The 20-minute workouts presented in these pages will give you the most efficient results in the shortest time. I believe that no time spent on Yoga is lost. If the 20 minutes of Yoga practice you give to yourself are full of your best attention, and if you practice every day, I know that it will work for you. You will start to feel stronger in just a week or two, and you will soon be using your new strength, confidence, and power to achieve your goals.

An Overview of the 20-Minute Workout

BREATHING: THE FIRST 2 MINUTES

To make your 20 minutes count, you have to shift as quickly as possible from your normal, everyday, outward-directed state of mind to a quieter, inward-directed state. Changing your breath pattern is the fastest way to do this, because the breath is a bridge between the outer and inner worlds. Changing your breathing pattern changes your thought pattern. This section starts with 2 seated breathing exercises, the first to loosen any stiffness in your lower back and the other to lengthen your breath and make it smoother. Then you stand up and continue breathing rhythmically to an 8-count breath. This is a transition between breathing for its own sake and breathing as a part of each Yoga exercise.

WARMING UP: 2 MINUTES

This section is a series of small movements designed to let your

WHERE YOGA CAME FROM

No one really knows when Yoga began, but its origins certainly predate written history. Yoga's roots can be traced back to the Aryan culture and possibly even before that. There is a common misconception that Yoga is rooted in Hinduism; even most dictionaries incorrectly state this in their definition of Yoga. If anything, Hinduism has incorporated Yoga into its religious thought, rather than the other way around. There are no beliefs or creeds that are prescribed by Yoga or followed by every Yoga practitioner, and so Yoga cannot be attached to any particular religion. My students have come from a wide variety of religious backgrounds.

The formal techniques of Yoga are based on the collective experiences of many individuals over many thousands of years; but even so, the emphasis is always on individual experience. You will never have exactly the same experience as anyone else, even when you are practicing exactly the same techniques, because your body and your mind are unlike anyone else's. Yoga encourages a scientific approach of observation and experimentation.

body know that you are beginning to exercise. The circulatory system is gently stimulated, and you begin to stretch the large muscle groups. No matter how strenuous your exercise routine, your warm-up period should always be gentle and slow.

EXERCISE: 8 MINUTES

Each Yoga exercise, or *asan*, has a particular effect on the body and mind. The exercises presented in this workout have been chosen because they represent a balance of effects on the body and mind, and because they will help you achieve the greatest benefit in the shortest time. The positions or movements included in this portion of the workout are presented in sequence, so there is as little extraneous movement between

positions as possible. This will help keep you focused on the routine.

RELAXATION AND MEDITATION: 8 MINUTES

Relaxation and meditation are taught in a lying-down position for the greatest comfort in the beginning. Later, when your back is stronger and your hips and knees more limber, you can try a seated position for meditation. The complete relaxation procedure teaches you how to relax at will. The purpose of meditation is to learn how to practice and enjoy stillness, inside and out.

That's the 20-minute workout. The remainder of this book shows you how to vary the workout for different stages in your life, physical conditions, or schedules.

Yoga for the Varieties of Your Life

WANT A MORE CHALLENGING WORKOUT?

If you've practiced Yoga before, or if you want to try a more strenuous workout, Chapter 6, "The 20-Minute Challenge," will teach you more intensive breathing techniques and exercises. Intensity in Yoga, however, is measured not just in physical strength, flexibility, or stamina, but primarily in attention and concentration. You'll find that the techniques in this chapter challenge you in more ways than one.

YOGA AND WOMEN'S ISSUES

The suggestions and special workouts in Chapter 7 can help women understand and cope better with the many changes that take place in their bodies at different times in their lives.

PMS (premenstrual syndrome) is a problem for about half of all women; sometimes a regular exercise program can make all the difference between suffering with days of incapacitation every month or sailing through with minimal discomfort. This 20-minute workout is designed especially to relax you at those times.

Pregnancy is a time to learn to be healthy, happy, and relaxed—the best way to welcome a happy baby into the family. During pregnancy, it is not advisable to do most Yoga exercises, but after the first trimester, a few gentle exercises that limber the hips and relax the spine, plus the daily benefits of breathing, relaxation, and meditation techniques, will do wonders for releasing tension and increasing your well-being. Many women have found that Yoga breathing exercises help make their labor and delivery experience easier. Remember to check all exercises with your doctor.

Menopause is dreaded by some, welcomed by others. About three-quarters of all women experience some menopausal symptoms. Yoga as part of a regular fitness program can help reduce the severity of many symptoms. The techniques included in this special 20-minute workout for menopause will balance the changes happening in your body and mind, and help you develop an attitude that looks forward, not back.

YOGA FOR TONING AND SHAPING AND TO BALANCE A SPORTS WORKOUT

Yoga is an all-around fitness program that gradually tones and shapes the body. Though it won't take off inches as fast as more vigorous exercise, Yoga will improve your posture, increase your willpower, and help you feel better about yourself as you follow a weight-loss program. You'll feel more attractive while you diet, and you'll find out that you can be happy while being self-disciplined. The 20-minute workout in the first part of Chapter 8 builds strength and stamina.

The second part of Chapter 8 offers some specific suggestions for adding a different dimension to sports and other forms of exercise. The 20-minute workout in this chapter improves concentration and stamina, and, because many sports programs emphasize weight training and aerobics that build muscle tissue rather than stretching it, the Yoga workout will add necessary flexibility.

WHEN YOU'RE AWAY FROM HOME

Your workplace can be either an obstacle course or a refuge when it comes to daily Yoga practice. If you habitually feel anxious and harried during your workday, try taking 20 minutes off and giving yourself a refreshing Yoga break. Chapter 9 includes a 20-minute workout that you can do at your desk, plus some ideas for using Yoga as a formidable reentry technique any time you've been away from home.

The demands of travel, including the stresses of strange surroundings, new people, and a different schedule, tend to push daily practice to the background. But it's never more important to make time for Yoga! Learning to adjust to change is a quality that will make the practice of Yoga (and every other aspect of life) much easier. What better opportunity to test your powers of flexibility than adapting to a new environment? Chapter 9 includes some suggestions for taking your workout with you when you're away from home.

SPECIAL HEALTH ISSUES

If you must modify the exercise segment of your workout due to back and neck problems, high blood pressure, recent injuries, convalescence, asthma, or recovery from addiction, Chapter 10 presents several modified routines. In addition to floor exercises, these include exercises that can be done in bed or in a chair.

GETTING THE MOST FROM YOUR WORKOUT

After the newness wears off, some people have trouble sticking with daily practice. Chapter 11 offers some helpful hints for avoiding boredom in your daily workout. The section "10 Ways to Be Your Own Best Friend" discusses a different way to look at ethical guidelines, and why practice of these principles can be an important component of reaching your goals in your 20-minute Yoga workout.

Yoga and Stress

A majority of my students initially decide to take a Yoga class in order to help themselves handle stress. We've all heard so much about stress in the last decade that the word has practically become a cliché. But whatever you call it, the effects are still there. How do all the different parts of you react when the world throws you a fastball? Do you feel anxious, fearful, grouchy, physically ill, nervous? Do you shake, tap your foot, breathe faster, click your pen, doodle? Do you shout, cry, hide, fight? Or do you reach for a cigarette, a drink, or a pill?

Any technique you employ to deal with stress is not, of course, designed to remove the source of the stress itself, but to help you change the way your body and mind *react* to stressors. Stress is a problem only when it becomes trapped. Yoga has gained a solid reputation for helping to release the negative stress reactions that grind down our health and well-being and prevent us from becoming as healthy and powerful as we could be. Practicing the 20-minute Yoga workout every day will give you the tools to use the positive qualities of stress for dynamic change.

By far the most useful and effective techniques for releasing stress reactions are breathing exercises, which protect the heart as well as calm the mind. Chapter 2 presents a complete discussion of why and how breathing works. Because of the concentrated breathing techniques included in your 20-minute workout, you may find that you automatically start to breathe differently at other times of the day. Encourage yourself to breathe deeply and completely, as often as you think about it, for an instant stress-reduction strategy.

Before You Start

Here are some general guidelines to help you get the most from your 20-minute workout:

1 *Check with your doctor* before beginning any new exercise program. Take this book with you and ask if there is anything you should avoid, especially if you have a chronic condition such as a neck or back problem.

2 *Be a friend to your body.* Don't overdo, especially if you haven't exercised in a long time. The idea is for all the parts of you to work together, instead of fighting each other. Don't let your mind ask your body to do something that will injure it.

3 *Set aside a time when you won't be interrupted.* The time of day doesn't matter so much as practicing every day. Many people find the morning hours quieter and more conducive to practice, but if you're not a "morning person," try it when you come home from work or just before going to bed. If you've scheduled your Yoga practice time for after work, take a bath or shower first to relax your muscles and wash off the cares of the day. Make conscious reentry a part of your Yoga workout.

4 *Find a large towel, a mat, or a blanket* that you use only for Yoga practice, and that is only for your own use. This will help you set a mood for practicing daily.

5 *Wear the same clothes* every day for Yoga practice; this will also help to get you in the mood to practice.

HOW TO PRACTICE YOGA HAPPILY EVERY DAY

The key to keeping up with any regular, disciplined practice is to enjoy it. Maybe the word "enjoy" is not altogether correct, because the word usually implies extreme happiness. For me, the concept of enjoyment has a deeper meaning—the idea of confident discovery. Every experience is a chance to learn something new. To a mystic, enjoyment would mean openness to change; the opposite of enjoyment, suffering, would mean being closed off from the opportunity to change. Anything that enhances your enjoyment of Yoga should be encouraged.

When you start practicing the 20-minute workout, keep a record of how you feel when you practice and of how you feel when you don't practice. Some people find it helpful to post a chart on the refrigerator or some other spot where they can see it and update it every day. Noticing your feelings about what you are doing will keep you interested in what happens next.

6 *Find one or more small, firm cushions* for the seated breathing techniques; you will also use these later when you move on to a seated meditation practice. Don't try to "tough it out" by sitting without support under your hips—it's not worth it! You'll only have to work harder to ignore the signals of fatigue and stiffness that your back will be sending you after a few minutes, and you won't be able to concentrate fully on the techniques. Use these cushions only for Yoga.

7 *Avoid practicing on a full stomach,* but a light snack before you begin is fine, especially if you practice right after work when you're prob- ably hungry. Avoid caffeine for an hour or two before practicing.

8 *Never practice Yoga under the influence of alcohol or recreational drugs.* If you are taking medication for psychiatric reasons, ask your doctor if there are any techniques you should avoid.

9 *Read the complete instructions* for each technique first, noting any cautions and hints. Sometimes it helps to practice in front of a mir- ror until you learn the exercises. After you've learned the correct movements and breathing, howev- er, your attention should be direct- ed inward, to how you feel as you do the exercise, and eventually to stillness, as in meditation.

Joining the Parts

The spirit of creativity that inspired the earliest practitioners of Yoga is exactly the attitude you can develop as you begin to prac- tice. Watch your body, breath, and mind. Notice how you feel with every movement, every breath, every thought. Pay attention to all the parts of yourself.

There are so many aspects to a

human being—physical, mental, emotional, creative, intuitive, vital, reactive, perceptive—the list goes on and on. Yoga is bringing together all the various parts of yourself in harmony so they work together, instead of fighting each other. Yoga means union with yourself—the solidification of who you are and the ability to put your full strength exactly where you want it, in confidence and happiness.

How to Use This Book

The first presentation of each technique includes a list of benefits, full instructions, and one or more photographs. In most cases, benefits and photos are not repeated if the technique is used in workout variations later in the book; the technique is listed with modified instructions, and you are referred back to the original presentation for benefits and illustrations.

2

BREATHING: THE FIRST 2 MINUTES

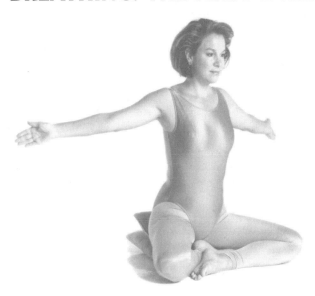

Your 20-minute workout starts with breathing exercises to begin the process of concentrating your energies inward. In order for the workout to be effective, your full attention must be there. Breathing helps to channel your attention from many different directions into one direction. It focuses and concentrates your attention in a very short time because of the close connection between the breath and the mind.

The strength of the body depends on breath. Breath is the bridge to consciousness and also the pathway to the superconsciousness of meditation. Breathing technique has always been important in the tradition of Yoga practice. My teacher, the great Lakshmanjoo, said that even if you are unable to do formal breathing techniques, "just watching the breath every moment will take you inside."

Slow Down, Detach, and Focus

In your 2 minutes of breathing exercises, you need to change your pace, release any stress reactions that are being carried by your body and mind, and turn your attention inward.

SLOW DOWN

No matter how organized your life, the demands of stress are always there. Even if you have learned how to see stress as a challenge rather than as a threat, the symptoms still exist. Pressure, anxiety, excitement, anticipation, heightened awareness, feeling pulls and pushes from all directions—these are all common emotional stress reactions. Among the many physical reactions are a rapid heartbeat, increased respiration, and muscle tension. Whether positive or negative, symptoms such as these cause hardship on the body by keeping it in a constant state of readiness for action (the "fight or flight" response). When things seem to be happening so fast that you feel out of control, it's time to regroup. Your 20-minute workout is designed to help release your reactions to stress, and the breathing techniques are the most efficient part of the workout for this task.

Yoga breathing techniques help you slow down long enough to get a grip on what's happening around you and within you. Though it seems paradoxical, the way to "get a grip" is to "let go." By forgetting everything and concentrating on the breath, your mind feels refreshed and rested, and you can go back into life with anticipation instead of dread, meeting all events knowing that your strength comes from within.

DETACH

The breathing techniques in your 20-minute workout will get you back to a steady state as quickly as possible with the minimum disruption. Breathing is your best, most efficient, most portable, most effective tool for doing this. You'll detach from the harsh cycle of reaction that has most of us ricocheting off one event after another all day long, like the steel ball in a pinball machine. Breathing techniques keep you from dwelling on the past or worrying about the future; instead, you learn to rest and be happy in the present moment.

FOCUS

Breath is the link between the inner and outer worlds. Breath is so closely tied to mood that you can actually change how you feel by changing your breath. Start to breathe faster, and you become charged up and outwardly directed; breathe slower, and you become more concentrated and inwardly directed.

When you do a breathing exercise, in order to focus more completely, think of the *breath breathing you* instead of you doing the breathing. Obviously, you don't have to tell your body when and how to breathe; it does so automatically. So now think of observing the breath so closely that you become one with it; your thought simply floats on the breath, and, in the process, both your mind and your body become more relaxed and quieter.

Physical Benefits of Breathing Practice

Regular practice of breathing techniques protects the heart and can help to reduce blood pressure, especially in combination with Yoga exercises and meditation. It does this by releasing muscle tension in the autonomic nervous system, which controls the con-

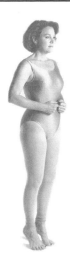

PRANA

Prana is a Sanskrit word that is often translated as "breath." For Yoga practitioners, it has a more subtle meaning—closer to "life." Prana means not just the outward manifestation of respiration but the subtle support of breath; in other words, *where breath comes from.* Before you feel the breath physically, a signal is sent from somewhere in your brain to your physical breathing apparatus that says it is time to breathe. That signal comes from *prana,* the vital life force that flows throughout the body, affecting its organs and functions in new ways, different from the way you ordinarily think of your daily functioning. Respiration is only one of the manifestations of this vital energy. *Prana* can be depleted by depression, a poor diet, and drugs; it can be replenished by rest, meditation, breathing exercises, and proper food. Connecting with or increasing *prana* makes you sparkle.

traction and relaxation of smooth muscles such as the heart and blood vessel walls. Breathing also can relieve insomnia, by relaxing the body and reducing the activity of the mind. If you have trouble sleeping, breathing exercises will help you to achieve peaceful, natural sleep without drugs or alcohol. Athletes use breathing exercises to increase strength and endurance and to be sure the muscles get oxygen to replenish stores depleted through exertion.

Helpful Hints

1 *Always breathe in and out through your nose* (unless you must breathe through your mouth for medical reasons). In other forms of exercise, the forced exhalation through pursed lips helps to expel air more quickly; for a beginner in Yoga, the point in breathing exercises is not to move air quickly but to relax, focus, and concentrate the mind. This can be accomplished much better by slowing down the movement of the breath.

If you find that one nostril is blocked and you can't breathe evenly, there is a simple technique for opening it. Make a fist and apply pressure in the armpit of the side that is *open* (the nerves that govern your left nostril, for instance, are located on the *right* side of your body) or lie on your side (again, the side that is open) for a few minutes.

2 *Focus your attention on the sound of the breath.* By closing your throat just slightly, you will notice a steamlike sound, not unlike the sound of a shell held up to your ear at the beach. You will feel it at the back of your throat first, instead of through the front of your nostrils, and it will feel cool. Focusing on the sound of the breath is the fastest way to become more concentrated. Closing your eyes also helps. Another aid is wax earplugs, available at any drugstore —the kind that swimmers use. Knead the wax in your hands to

soften it, and press it over the ear opening. If you push it too far in, you'll be distracted by all the sounds your body makes—the blood pulsing, joints creaking, and so on. By just covering the ear opening, you'll intensify the sound of the breath so you can concentrate better, and also remove the distraction of outside noises. If you live on a busy street or feel distracted by other activities going on in your home, use the earplugs for your meditation, too.

3 *Give yourself time to warm up.* Yes, there has to be a warm-up period even in breathing. This means that your first breaths will be shorter, and they will gradually lengthen with practice. Each breathing segment suggests a certain number of repetitions. Start with relatively short breaths and gradually extend the length with each repetition.

4 *Breathing is not a competitive sport!* Although the idea should be to gradually extend the breath to longer cycles, the goal in this practice is not simply longer breath for its own sake; instead, try to notice how you feel while you're breathing, and learn how to use the breath to change how you feel and to answer the needs of the body.

5 *Find a comfortable seated position.* There is nothing more important in breathing exercises than establishing a position that you can hold for several minutes without strain. Ideally, this would be a seated position where your back is straight. If you are limber enough, sit on the floor with your hips elevated on one or more cushions. Sit cross-legged on the edge of the cushions so your pelvis tilts for-

ward slightly and your knees touch the floor (A). If your knees are still elevated even with the cushions, try straddling the cushions (B). You can also do breathing exercises very successfully while sitting on the edge of a bed or chair (C, next page). The same rule applies—hips higher than knees—so you may have to tuck your toes under to find the correct position for breathing. If you have a bad back, or for some other reason can't find a comfortable seated position, you may do your breathing lying down with cushions under your legs to take pressure off your lower back. Don't use

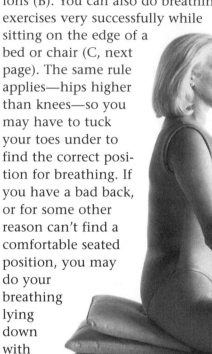

A

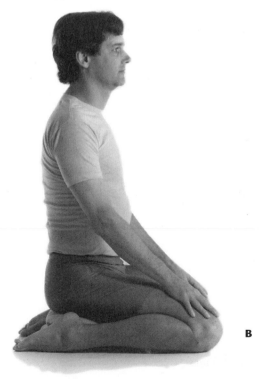

B

a pillow under your head; remember, no matter what position you end up in, your spine should remain straight, and that includes the neck. Try not to have any pressure on the back of the head or neck. If your floor is hard, lie on a foam mat or a folded blanket.

The reason it is so important to find the proper position is that when your hips are elevated, your lower back tilts forward slightly and your stomach muscles can relax, allowing you to take fuller, longer, and deeper breaths. If you try to maintain a seated position without a relaxed back and stomach, you won't be able to take a full breath.

6 *Keep your arms away from your rib cage.* Many people are unsure what to do with their arms and hands. There is no need to hold your hands in any special position. The main point to remember is to keep the rib cage free to expand to its fullest when you breathe in. Put your hands on your knees, on your hips, or on your stomach. Never breathe with your hands in your lap because you won't be able to expand your rib cage completely.

7 *Don't hold your breath at any time.* Make the transition between inhalation and exhalation, and vice versa, smooth and quiet.

C

The Breathing Techniques

Arched Breath

Limbers the muscles used for breathing; limbers the spine

Sit on your feet with knees together, or take any other comfortable seated position. Place your hands on your knees. Start by breathing in (through your nose, remember) and arching your back forward, stretching the entire spine from the tailbone to the back of the neck (D). Breathe out and round your back in the opposite direction, tucking your head (E). Coordinate the breath with the movement so you're breathing the whole time you're moving. Breathe as fully and completely as possible.

Repetitions: 3-5

D

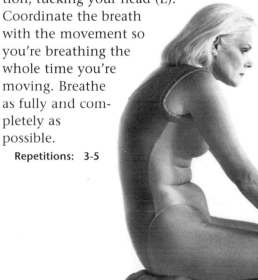

E

THE PHYSIOLOGY OF BREATH

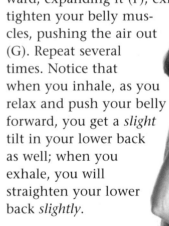

Strictly speaking, the lungs don't do your breathing for you; rather, the muscles surrounding the lungs do it. Breathing involves quite a few muscles, and most people use only a few of them. The diaphragm is the most important muscle. It stretches from the lower front rib cage to the midback. It is flat and round. This is where the signal to breathe first comes. In order to breathe in, the diaphragm expands downward, causing the lungs to expand. When this happens, the pressure inside the lungs decreases, and air is pulled in from outside to compensate. In breathing out, the reverse happens: the diaphragm first contracts (pulls up), increasing pressure in the lungs, then air is expelled to compensate. Other muscles between each rib help to expand or contract the lungs by expanding or contracting the rib cage. Still other muscles across the stomach, sides, and back— vertical, horizontal, and diagonal—also aid respiration.

Complete Breath (Seated)

Focuses the mind and exercises all the respiratory muscles

Because this exercise requires some coordination of body parts, I've divided it into 3 sections: learning the exercise, practicing the exercise, and timing.

Learning the exercise Sit in your most comfortable seated position. In the Complete Breath, you will be using the muscles of your stomach and lower back, rib cage, and upper chest. Your head, neck, and upper back should remain straight.

For the first stage—the stomach and the lower back—start by placing your hands on your belly. Inhale and push your belly forward, expanding it (F); exhale and tighten your belly muscles, pushing the air out (G). Repeat several times. Notice that when you inhale, as you relax and push your belly forward, you get a *slight* tilt in your lower back as well; when you exhale, you will straighten your lower back *slightly*.

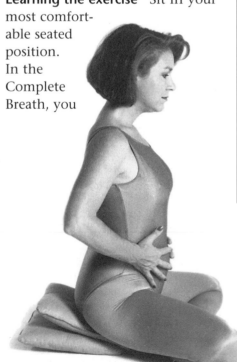

F

G

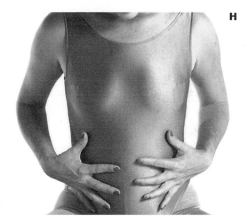

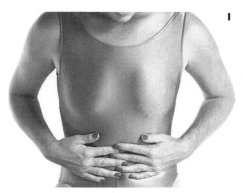

For the second stage of the exercise, the ribs, place your hands higher so you can feel your ribs. Your fingers should be just touching. Inhale and expand the ribs (H), noticing that your fingers are pulled apart slightly; exhale and contract your ribs (I), noticing that your fingers are touching again. Put the first two stages together: as you inhale, relax and expand the belly, then expand the ribs. As you exhale, contract the ribs and then tighten the belly to push out the last of the air.

The third stage, expanding the chest, is a more subtle movement. After you've expanded your belly and your ribs, your lungs will be nearly full. At the top of the inhalation, expand the top of your chest just slightly, to get the last of the air in; your shoulders lift just a little. Don't strain. As you begin to exhale, relax your shoulders first, then the ribs, then the belly.

Practicing the exercise As you begin to *inhale*, relax your belly and push it forward, then expand the ribs, and finally expand the chest and feel the shoulders lift slightly. When you *exhale*, let the chest relax first, then let the ribs relax, and finally tighten your belly muscles as you push out the last of the air. Keep inhalation and exhalation equal. Focus on the sound of the breath.

Repetitions: 5-10

Use your hands, if necessary, to guide you until you've mastered the mechanics of the Complete Breath. Remember to breathe through your nose. Breathe in from the bottom up; breathe out from the top down. At first, you'll be using all your attention just in learning the pattern of breath. After you've been practicing for a while, your mind may start to drift while you're breathing; gently bring your attention back to the sound of the breath.

Timing The Complete Breath is designed to be practiced in even lengths—breathing out for the same length of time that you breathe in. This is one of the ways that it creates a balanced mind. If you've never practiced breathing exercises or stretched your breath before, you probably will start out at about 5–8 seconds in, 5–8 seconds out. You'll probably notice that you can naturally breathe out longer than you can breathe in. Most people observe this pattern. In this case, you'll need to shorten the exhalation to match the inhalation; if you try to stretch the inhalation, you won't be able to sustain it for very long. If you have a clock or watch with a second hand, you can check the timing of your breath. If not, just count to yourself, "one thousand one, one thousand two," and so on. But don't time your breath every day. Remember, the most important aspect of breath is the *sound*.

Try practicing the Complete Breath whenever you think of it—at the office, in the car, while you're waiting in line at the grocer—and notice how you feel while you're breathing. Does the breath change how you feel?

Standing 8-Count Breath

Suffuses the body with oxygen and energy; creates a beautiful glow

If you've been sitting cross-legged for the Complete Breath, stretch your legs out in front of you, checking your joints and muscles for any tension before you stand up. Now, standing with feet parallel, take a deep breath and stretch toward the ceiling; breathe out and relax. Now close your eyes and continue the Complete Breath, this time counting to 8 as you inhale, and again as you exhale. If you run out of breath before you get to 8, start by counting to 5. Use the same procedure of breathing in from the belly up to the chest, and breathing out from the chest down.

Repetitions: 3

3

WARMING UP: 2 MINUTES

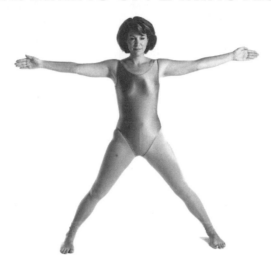

The 2 minutes of breathing techniques that open your 20-minute workout start to change your outlook to one that is more inner-directed. You feel a little less hurried, less pressured, less tense. You catch a glimpse of something timeless that supports and sustains you. Your mind begins to move away from daily cares to prepare for meditation.

In this next segment of your 20-minute workout, you will begin to transfer that feeling to your body with slow movements that start a process of relaxing and letting go of tension and anxieties about the day past or the day to come. To get the most from your warm-up sequence, keep bringing your attention back to the present moment. Ask yourself "What am I feeling?" during and after each exercise.

The warm-up sequence is designed to begin to loosen the joints, get your blood moving, gently begin to stretch your large muscles, and, most important, get in touch with your body. Your body is your friend in Yoga, not your enemy. Learn to work with it, not against it. Don't push or strain. Don't force any movement. There is no need to do everything perfectly the first time. If you are practicing first thing in the morning, you'll be somewhat stiff; work with it, not against it. There should be a sense of letting go while warming up, where you not only set the stage for the more vigorous part of your workout but also take pleasure in getting to know your body better. These small movements allow you to pay attention to and take care of any problems before you go into the slightly more strenuous movements of *asans* (Yoga exercises), so you don't injure yourself. Warming up properly helps to remove fear from the body.

LEARN TO LET TENSION FLOW THROUGH

Tension is a problem only if it is trapped. Otherwise, it is a positive force that energizes and motivates us to act. We block our capabilities by refusing to recognize stress and tension and allow them expression. They get blocked in their passage through the body and cause many physical and emotional problems. Nonviolent expression lets stress and tension flow through and then leave without the toxic residue of muscle tightness, joint pain, and impaired breathing. Yoga prepares the channels in the body so that stress and tension can be expressed with strength, confidence, and health.

Warming up also brings mental concentration into balance with what's happening in the body. Most people simply "fall" into concentration without awareness; the warm-up process shows you how to bring concentration simultaneously to both mind and body, so that you get the best effect from your 20-minute workout.

Warm-ups work on the major muscle groups, especially the areas most likely to be stiff or tight. Because the health, strength, and limberness of the spinal column are so important in Yoga, the warm-up sequence includes several movements that start limbering all sections of the spinal column. Getting your circulation moving increases body temperature and relaxes your muscles.

Starting with warm-ups gently coaxes your body into more vigorous movements. Many people rush into an exercise routine thinking, "I'm going to do this no matter what, and my body just has to keep up. That's all there is to it."

Your body is not a robot that you can push around indefinitely without care for how it feels. The body has its own consciousness, its own wants and needs, and its own feelings. It will not always function perfectly, no matter how much you want it to, and if you force it, you'll just cause it to dig in its heels and sulk—or give up. You should never push your body into a strenuous exercise; take time to observe what your body can do and how it feels when it does each movement. By starting slowly, you persuade your body that moving feels good and that it can move through some stiffness without pain or injury. As your body becomes more confident, you can add more vigorous movements easily.

Some days, if you are really in a rush (days when you may not have even 20 minutes for a full workout), just do a few warm-ups. Take a 20-*second* break in the middle of the day to stretch a little. Use your coffee break for a rest break for your body. Just those few exercises will make a big difference in how you feel, and they will maintain the momentum of daily practice that is really essential in Yoga.

Learning to Listen to Your Body

Sometimes we treat our bodies like automatons. We expect them to work, and we feel betrayed when they become ill, develop a pain, or show signs of growing old. We generally take our bodies for granted. In Yoga it's important to learn to listen to your body, which simply means paying attention. Treat your body like a child. Learn to recognize its moods. Put yourself in your body's position. Act as if you were your physical consciousness. When you get really good at listening to your body, you will be able to create your own exercise routine simply by asking your body what it needs and wants to do that day. When you are listening to your body, remember that it expresses itself in feelings. It feels fatigue, for instance, or it feels a tightness in the back of the legs, or perhaps it feels afraid of twisting in a certain way. Choose your exercises to make the body happy.

On a day when you have a little more time to practice, try this exercise: Close your eyes and pay attention exclusively to your physical body, as if it were a separate person standing in front of you. Notice your face. Does any part of your face feel tight? Check the muscles around your eyes and your jaw. Check your forehead. Do the same with your shoulders, your back, your knees, and your feet. Listen for feelings of tightness or looseness, tension or relaxation, vulnerability or strength—and any other feeling that comes to mind. How are those feelings affecting you?

Now think of all the different exercises you know. Visualize yourself doing some of them. Ask

THE IMPORTANCE OF DAILY PRACTICE

Make the commitment to practice *something* every day—even if that something is just the 2-minute warm-up or breathing segment from your regular 20-minute workout. In Yoga, the effect is cumulative; its force builds in your body and mind over time according to the attention you give it. When you practice every day, you eventually create an unbroken river of health, steadiness, and support in your unconscious that makes you powerful and happy.

THE SOUND OF THE BREATH

If you find your attention wandering while you are exercising, concentrate on the sound of your breath going in and out. It's a steamlike sound that you make by closing your throat slightly. Make the sound even and smooth, and let it fill your head. Breathe as loudly as you can without straining. The sound of the breath will focus your mind and greatly intensify your workout experience.

your body what it would like to do. Does it need to bend? Does it need to stretch? Does it want to do something aerobic? If you've never tried this, and if you are a sedentary sort of person, you might think that this exercise would always result in your body asking to go back to sleep! But if you listen closely, and check with your body regularly, you'll discover your body asking for the things it really wants and needs, like exercise and good food, in addition to enough rest and care.

Helpful Hints

This sequence should take you about 2 minutes, allowing for a short rest after the Side Stretch and for a hold of at least 20 seconds in the Full Bend Hold.

Do each exercise at half capacity at first. Though the techniques in the 8-minute exercise segment are usually done in threes, warm-ups can be repeated several times. The idea is to loosen up slowly, so that by the time you go into your main exercise routine, you're more focused and your body is more relaxed and ready. Be sure to do the same number of repetitions on each side to balance the body.

The Warm-up Sequence

Shoulder Roll

Loosens shoulder joints and upper back muscles

Keeping your arms loose at your sides, lift your shoulders and roll them forward, down, back, and up in a smooth circle (A). Continue rolling forward 3 or 4 times, then reverse and roll back, down, forward, and up several times. Keep arms and hands loose and eyes open. Breathe normally. The purpose of this exercise is to loosen the muscles of the upper back and shoulders, where a lot of tension is trapped. If you work at a desk much of the day, and especially if you do a lot of work at a keyboard, do this exercise several times a day to keep from building up tension in your upper back and neck.

Repetitions: 4-5 in each direction

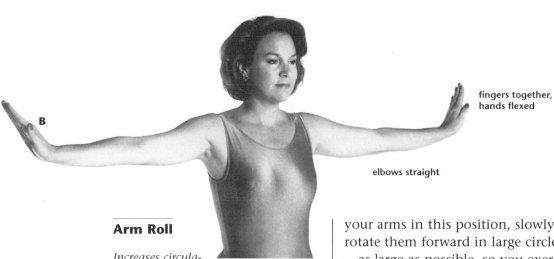

fingers together, hands flexed

elbows straight

B

Arm Roll

Increases circulation; strengthens back and shoulders; improves range of motion of shoulders; limbers upper back, chest, and midback muscles

Hold your arms straight out to your sides with elbows straight. Face your hands away from you, as if you were stopping traffic on either side of you (B). Holding your arms in this position, slowly rotate them forward in large circles —as large as possible, so you exercise the full range of motion of your shoulder joints. Keep the fingers stretched back. Do 3 or 4 large circles in each direction, then do a few smaller circles in each direction. Let your arms relax, and shake them out.

Repetitions: 3-4 in each direction (large circles); 4-5 in each direction (small circles)

Head Roll

Limbers neck muscles and cervical spine; improves circulation in throat

Stand with arms at your sides or hands on your hips. Keep your shoulders relaxed throughout, breathe normally, and keep your eyes open. Start by bending your head forward and relaxing the back of your neck (C). Slowly rotate your head to one side so your ear is over your shoulder (D). Continue rolling around and tilt your head back carefully (E), then over to the other shoulder, and back to the

C

D

ear over shoulder

shoulders relaxed

E

front. Repeat 3 or more times in each direction. Caution: Do not do this exercise if you have a disk problem in your neck. With your doctor's permission, you may substitute a simple and slow side-to-side and up-and-down motion without the roll and without tilting your head back.

Repetitions: 3 in each direction

Elbow Twist

Limbers spine; improves respiration and posture

Stand with your feet a few inches apart. Extend your arms, bending them at the elbow, and place one hand on top of the other. Breathe in, straightening your spine, and breathe out as you twist slowly

around to one side, leading with one elbow (F). Twist as far around as you can, feeling the stretch all along your spine from your tailbone to the back of your neck. Stretch your eyes and facial muscles by looking back over your shoulder as far as possible. Breathe in and return to the front, then breathe out and twist to the opposite side. If everything in your back and neck feels fine, you can increase the speed of this exercise slightly for a couple of repetitions.

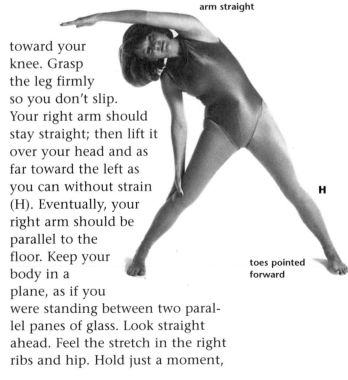

Repetitions: 3 in each direction

Side Stretch

Limbers back, legs, hips; limbers intercostal muscles (rib cage); improves respiration and balance

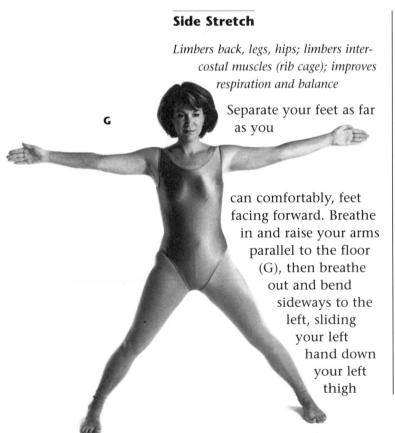

Separate your feet as far as you can comfortably, feet facing forward. Breathe in and raise your arms parallel to the floor (G), then breathe out and bend sideways to the left, sliding your left hand down your left thigh toward your knee. Grasp the leg firmly so you don't slip. Your right arm should stay straight; then lift it over your head and as far toward the left as you can without strain (H). Eventually, your right arm should be parallel to the floor. Keep your body in a plane, as if you were standing between two parallel panes of glass. Look straight ahead. Feel the stretch in the right ribs and hip. Hold just a moment,

arm straight

H

toes pointed forward

then breathe in and come back up to the first position with arms outstretched. Breathe out and bend toward the right. Repeat twice more on each side. Make this a smooth, easy movement; it's easy to overdo and strain by reaching too far down the leg. Keep both knees straight.

Repetitions: 3 on each side

Full Bend Variation

Improves posture; limbers shoulder joints and upper back vertebrae; improves respiration

Clasp your hands behind your back and straighten your arms (I). If you can, lock your elbows as shown and press your palms together so your shoulder blades are squeezed together as tightly as possible. Breathe in, standing straight, then breathe out and bend forward, keeping your arms pulled back and away from your body (J). Keep

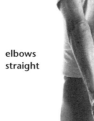

I

elbows straight

palms together

knees straight. Breathe in and straighten back to your starting position. If it is difficult to sustain the arms-locked position for all 3 repetitions, relax your arms, shake them out, and gently roll your head back and forth for a moment between each complete movement.

Repetitions: 3

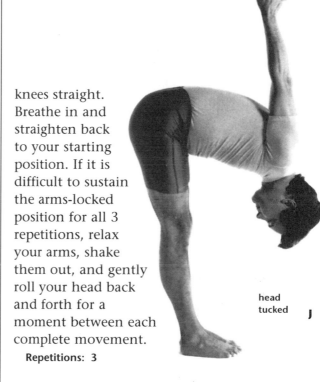

head tucked   J

Full Bend Hold

Releases tension in the upper back and neck; helps to reduce a large stomach

After your third Full Bend Variation, breathe out and come forward once again, but let your arms relax toward the floor (K). If you can reach the floor comfortably, let your fingers curl slightly. Go limp and relax, let your head hang so your

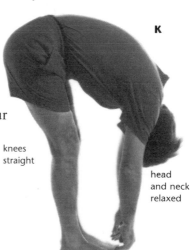

K

knees straight

head and neck relaxed

neck stretches out a bit, and relax your breath. Hold for several seconds, then slowly stand up. If your lower back is tight, don't hold as long.

Repetitions: 1

Leg Swing

Limbers hip joints; strengthens legs; improves balance

Put both hands on your hips. Lift your left leg in front of you, with the toes flexed and both knees straight (L), and then swing it to the back, keeping knees straight. Don't lean forward. Breathe normally.

Repetitions: 4-6 for each leg

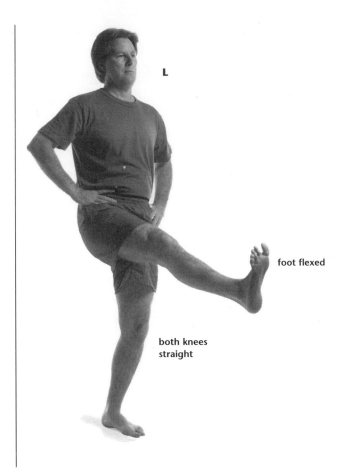

L

foot flexed

both knees straight

4

EXERCISE: 8 MINUTES

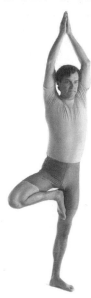

You'll experience this 8-minute segment as a workout for many different systems in your body and mind. Yoga exercises, or *asans*, are very efficient movements of the body and breath that affect your entire being. Some of the most obvious effects are described in the sections that follow.

Balance

Your physical sense of balance is enhanced by poses done on one leg at a time, or on toes, or on all fours. These poses also strengthen the leg and back muscles, and eyesight.

There is also the concept of balance between the two halves of the body—right and left. You've probably noticed that you favor one side of your body over the other when you're playing a sport or writing. That side is a little stronger and a little more coordinated than the other because you use it more often. Yoga exercises help equalize the two halves of the body by strengthening the central nervous system, which directs all parts of the body.

Then there is the difference between the two halves of your brain: the right brain, which takes primary responsibility for spatial, holistic, imaging, and mystical experiences, perceptions, and expressions; and the left brain, which takes primary responsibility for language, analysis, and verbal experiences, perceptions, and expressions. Yoga stimulates both sides of your brain and allows you to become much more aware of how you think and react, and what you feel, using the many wonderful resources of your whole mind.

Balance is also reflected in the relative weight we give to various aspects of our lives. If you are a workaholic, you probably are not balancing your job and personal life. Similarly, if you are constantly following the latest fad diet or exercising to exhaustion every day, you probably are not balanced in your concept of health maintenance. Because Yoga improves health, it motivates you to avoid extremes that could be self-destructive. Practicing Yoga regularly will teach you how to create a balanced mind and body that will support the choices you make in life.

Poise

How you stand, walk, and carry your body will change almost immediately. As Yoga exercises strengthen the postural muscles on either side of your spine and the abdominal muscles that help to support your lower back, and as they relax the upper back muscles that get tired so easily, you'll notice yourself standing taller and walking more fluidly. Stress shows itself very clearly in posture; Yoga helps you walk tall and strong.

Poise also has to do with mental presence. Your self-awareness will improve as you practice your workout, because you're becoming more knowledgeable about both your body and your mind. By paying attention to how you feel, you learn who you are and how to discover the source of your personal power.

Flow

Yoga exercises improve your body's circulation by stretching the major muscle groups, by increasing the elasticity of blood vessels, and by gently exercising the heart and lungs. At the same time, muscles are flooded with fresh oxygen and other nutrients, and the toxins and waste products that build up in the muscles are flushed out. Yoga exercises put gentle pressure on the glands and organs, improving the normal production and release of necessary hormones.

Yoga exercises increase energy flow. We all unconsciously tighten our physical body when we experience anxiety, fear, or other stressors. This physical and mental rigidity blocks not only happiness but also creativity; it takes a great deal of energy to maintain the rigid stance. Yoga exercises release the tightness, allowing energy to be released and renewed, and allowing creativity and productivity to bloom.

Flexibility

Yoga exercises stretch and limber the muscles, joints, and connective tissue. The stretches in your 20-minute workout form a well-balanced routine that increases the limberness and range of motion of all major joints and muscles. Because the spine is so important, most exercises affect the spine in some way. The range of movements includes forward bends, backward bends, side stretches, and twisting movements.

Flexibility of the mind is a quality that emerges from regular practice of Yoga. Yoga stimulates change; the ability to accept—and even celebrate—change is a very freeing quality. When you can see the tremendous energy that it takes to maintain a rigid, unchanging viewpoint, you may find that Yoga gives you the courage to release that energy and use it to visualize and achieve the health, happiness, and power that you want; this is the freedom of awareness that comes from flexibility in Yoga.

Strength

Yoga *asans* tone and strengthen all major muscle groups, especially the postural muscles and the muscles in the legs and stomach. Smooth muscles such as those of the heart and blood vessels are also strengthened by gentle exertion and pressure. The joints and bones are strengthened through gentle weight-bearing exercises and holding positions. You'll notice that all movements are slow and deliberate, so you gain maximum benefit from each efficient position.

Yoga builds mental and emotional strength by making you aware of the untapped source of support that is in your inner being. Yoga supports your need for consistency, rest, concentration, willpower, and purpose. Yoga builds self-confidence, enabling you to be the person you want to be. Strength of will often emerges from the feelings of freedom and possibility—the feeling that anything is possible; that no goal is unachievable. Often these feelings are constrained by the emotional tension that accompanies physical tension. While releasing physical tension, Yoga *asans* effect the release of emotional tension as well.

Imagination

People have an image of their bodies that grows more embedded over time as it is reinforced by the mind. This was illustrated very clearly to me in a class I taught several years ago. One of my students had recently lost quite a bit of weight. The room where I taught had desks and chairs piled up in the back of the room next to several pillars. One day I noticed this student coming in through one of the gaps between the furniture and a pillar; she squeezed herself sideways to get through, even though there was obviously plenty of room for her to walk through, facing forward, with no trouble. I asked her why she had come through sideways, and she said,

HOW YOGA *ASANS* GOT THEIR NAMES

You'll notice as you continue practicing that many Yoga *asans* are named for animals (such as the Tortoise Stretch). Some people think this is simply because the pose looks somewhat like that animal. This is only partially correct. The real reason has to do with why the exercises are performed in the first place. In the classical sense, Yoga *asans* are done not just for physical effects but also to understand and identify with the beautiful qualities of the animals, beings, and actions they are named for. When you perform the Sun Pose, for example, you think of the energizing, life-giving properties of the sun, without which all life on Earth would die. Your unconscious resonates with those qualities that are in your collective memory from earliest evolutionary times.

"Oh, I could never get through that small space; I'm too big." She had internalized her obesity to such an extent that now, even though she had lost so much weight, she still envisioned herself as heavy and large.

In Yoga, the capacity for fantasy can open the mind to new possibilities and changes that may be difficult to imagine. To use fantasy to best advantage, spend a few minutes every day imagining yourself the way you want to be. Create a strong picture in your mind, full of details, imagining the way you want to look, the way you want to act and react, and what you wish to achieve. This will steadily reinforce that picture of yourself in your unconscious mind, and eventually you'll see the results in your conscious life.

As you practice Yoga *asans*, imagine yourself performing each one perfectly. Even though your physical position may not match your mental image, the strength of your thought will give you the same benefits—both physical and mental—as the perfect position. If you are unable to practice Yoga *asans* due to injury or illness, do them in your mind, and the benefits will be there as well.

The Chemistry of Yoga *Asans*

Yoga *asans* stimulate the release of endorphins, the substances in the brain that cause us to feel pleasure. Any vigorous exercise will cause this physical effect, but regular practice of Yoga *asans* results in these feelings being sustained over time. The gentle but constant pressure on glands and organs in the various positions stimulates the production of hormones, and the improved circulation guarantees their distribution throughout the body and brain. The specific improvement in respiration produced by Yoga *asans* results in the brain receiving more oxygen more of the time.

The most pronounced mental change that occurs as a result of such sustained physical effects over time is noticed by most students within a few weeks of beginning daily practice. A combination of a more efficient and relaxed body, hormonal stimulation, more oxygen, and better rest and care means a greater and more constant feeling of well-being.

Helpful Hints

BREATHING IN YOGA *ASANS*

One of the most important instructions in practicing Yoga *asans* is to coordinate the body and breath. When an exercise asks you to breathe and move at the same time, try to match the movement to your breath, so you start breathing as you start to move, and when you stop moving, your breath is completely in or completely out. This increases the efficiency of the body's exchange of gases in the lungs, and also helps you concentrate on what you are doing. You won't be able to use the same three stages of breathing as in the Complete Breath, but try to breathe as completely as possible, focus on the sound of the breath coming from the back of your throat, and always breathe through your nose (see Chapter 2 for a review of these suggestions for better breathing).Concentrating on the sound of the breath is one way to keep your attention on what you are doing; your mind will tend to wander after you've learned the *asans* so well that you don't have to think about what to do next.

Usually, you will be instructed to breathe in as you straighten up, stretch, or otherwise expand your rib cage, and breathe out as you fold in half or compress your rib cage, which is a natural way to breathe that enhances the normal expansion and contraction of your lungs. Occasionally, you will be instructed to breathe in while you *compress* the body, in order to push oxygen and nutrients through the bloodstream, muscles, and organs more forcefully.

Because every exercise begins with an inhalation, start by exhaling completely. Then when you inhale, you'll be filling your lungs completely during the exercise.

PAY ATTENTION TO DETAILS

In Yoga *asans*, every position of every part of the body has meaning. Pay attention to instructions concerning such details as the position of your fingers, the angle of your head, where your eyes are focused, and the direction of your feet. Remember to relax any muscle that is not needed in the exercise. If you are instructed to hold a position, create the idea of relaxing *into* the position (see sidebar, "The *Asan* Point," page 61).

REST AS OFTEN AS NECESSARY

This 8-minute segment of your workout allows for two rests of approximately 1 minute each: the Baby Pose and the Corpse Pose. Don't hesitate to rest more often or longer if you feel the need. Remember, your workout should energize you, not tire you out. During your rest poses, think of going completely limp, like a rag doll. Let your breath relax completely back to a normal resting pattern. Survey your body quickly, paying special attention to the parts that tend to tighten up most: your jaw, your eyes, your shoulders, your stomach. Relax those spots. Then stop all mental conversation for several seconds while you rest your mind.

The *Asan* Routine

Before you start: Have near you a shawl or extra blanket with which to cover yourself, plus a pair of socks, so you can go straight into meditation after the *asan* routine without distractions and without getting chilled.

Standing Sun Pose

Improves functioning of digestive and circulatory systems; exercises heart and lungs; limbers and strengthens legs and back

Stand with feet parallel. Breathe out completely. Start to breathe in and raise your arms in a circle to the sides and over your head, palms together. Your breath should be all the way in. Look up at your hands (A).

stretch and look up

A

Now breathe out as you bend forward *from the waist* (B), keeping your back as straight as you can for as long as possible. Keep your head between your arms. When you're as far forward as possible, grasp your ankles, calves, or knees with both hands (get a good, firm grip) and bend your elbows slightly to pull your upper body toward your legs (C). Your breath should be completely out. Keep knees straight and tuck your head.

bend from waist

head between arms

Important: If you can't bend your elbows, you're grasping too far down your legs. Move your grip higher so you can bend your elbows; otherwise, you'll be pulling with your back muscles, which could strain your back. Be sure to use your arms to pull yourself down.

After holding for a few seconds with your breath

knees straight

B

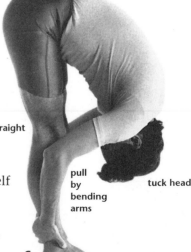

pull by bending arms

tuck head

C

out, release your legs and slowly come back up to a standing position, bringing your arms out to the sides and up in a circular motion. Stretch and look up with palms together (A), then breathe out and lower your arms to your sides in a final circle. Always move your arms in as wide a circle as you can in order to increase the expansion of the chest.

Repetitions: 3

Twisting Triangle

Increases flexibility and circulation in hips and lower back; strengthens hip joints and upper back; helps relieve depression

Separate your feet as far as you can comfortably (without losing your balance) and point your toes forward. Breathe in and raise your arms to the sides, parallel to the floor. Breathe out as you bend toward the left leg, grasp the *outside* of your left ankle (or calf) with your right hand, then turn your head so you are looking at your left hand, which should be pointed straight up, fingers curled and thumb toward you (D). Stare at your thumb. Pull slightly with your right hand to increase the stretch. Keep both knees straight.

Hold for a second or two, then breathe in and come back to your starting position, arms outstretched. Breathe out and repeat to the right leg.

Repetitions: 3 on each side

look at thumb

D   hand on outside of ankle   toes pointed forward

Bring your feet together and stand with eyes closed, body and breath relaxed, for a few seconds until your breath returns to normal.

Tree Pose

Improves posture, poise, balance, concentration, respiration; strengthens legs

Stare at one spot on the wall or floor in front of you (but keep your head straight). Breathing normally, slowly raise your right leg and place your right foot as high on the inside of your left leg as possible. Point the toes down and relax the leg; both these suggestions will help keep your foot from slipping down your leg. When you feel steady, exhale completely, then slowly breathe in and raise your arms over your head. Straighten your arms and place your palms together (E). Now relax your breath and hold the pose for 10 to 30 seconds. Watch for tightness in your stomach muscles, which will tense your breathing. Relax your breath throughout. Keep staring at one spot for balance. Hold for several seconds, then slowly lower arms and leg. Repeat with the other leg. If you have trouble balancing, practice this exercise standing next to a sturdy chair or the wall, and hold on with one hand. It's more important to relax your breath in this balance pose than to raise your arms overhead.

Repetitions: 1 on each side

arms as straight as possible

stare at one spot

breath relaxed

E

Baby Pose

Limbers and relaxes lower back; improves circulation to the brain and pelvic region; improves reproductive and digestive systems' functioning; improves respiration; reduces large stomach

Sit on your feet with knees together. Slowly bend forward so your head touches the floor. Let your arms rest at your sides with your elbows bent so they rest on the floor (F). This will relax your shoulders and neck. Your head can rest on the forehead or bridge of the nose. Wiggle around a bit to find the most comfortable position. Let your breath relax, and hold for at least a minute. If this position is not comfortable, try resting your head on folded arms; if that is still too uncomfortable, use this position as an exercise, hold it for only a few seconds, then lie down on your back to rest.

Repetitions: 1

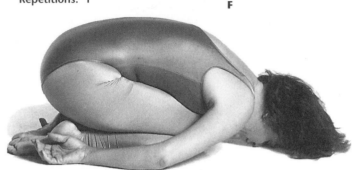

F

Cobra Pose

Improves functioning of digestive, respiratory, and reproductive systems; limbers and strengthens entire spine; strengthens eyesight; equalizes two sides of body; improves complexion

Lie on your stomach with legs together (those with occasional lower back trouble should separate the legs at first). Place your forehead on the floor and your palms underneath your shoulders, close to your body, so your elbows point up (G), not out to the sides. Breathe out completely, then start to breathe in as you curl first your head and eyes back as far as they will go, then your chest, and then your stomach. Keep your hipbones on the floor—this is not a push-up—and your arms slightly bent (unless you are *extremely* limber). Use your back muscles more than your arms. Hold for a few seconds at the top, with your breath in and eyes looking up through your forehead (H). Then start to breathe out and curl forward slowly, in reverse: your stomach curls down first, then your chest, and finally your head and eyes. Your eyes are the first part of your body to curl up and the last to curl down.

Repetitions: 3

Caution: This is a very powerful exercise and should not be done if you have had recent surgery, if you have an open cut anywhere on your body, or by women during the menstrual period.

G

look up

use back muscles

H

ankles together
if possible

HOW TO GET THE MOST EFFICIENT, RELAXED STRETCH

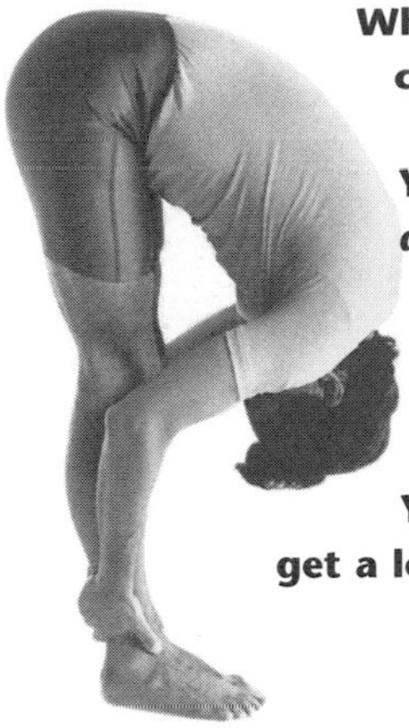

When you stretch a muscle nearly to its limit, its automatic reaction is to contract slightly, so that it doesn't tear. This is especially true when you bounce or stretch hard, as in some calisthenic-type exercise routines. In Yoga it's important always to stretch slowly and smoothly; most Yoga *asans* also incorporate a particular breathing pattern. Although in a beginning routine you should not hold a pose for more than a few seconds, you can accomplish a lot in those few seconds. When you are stretched to what you think is your limit, consciously relax *into* the stretch, and hold, breathing gently and stopping mental conversation. You'll find that the muscles will release themselves a bit more and you'll get a longer, more relaxed stretch without pain.

Tortoise Stretch

Improves circulation to pelvic region; stretches nerves and muscles in legs and ankles; limbers lower back; helps prevent prostate problems

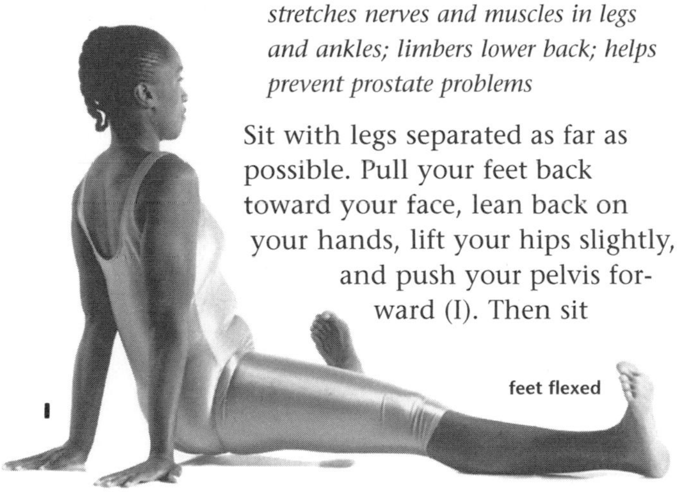

Sit with legs separated as far as possible. Pull your feet back toward your face, lean back on your hands, lift your hips slightly, and push your pelvis forward (I). Then sit

feet flexed

I

straight, rest your hands on your legs, and point your toes (J). Hold for a few seconds. Repeat twice more. Then, with feet pulled back again, breathe in and raise your arms in a circle over your head.

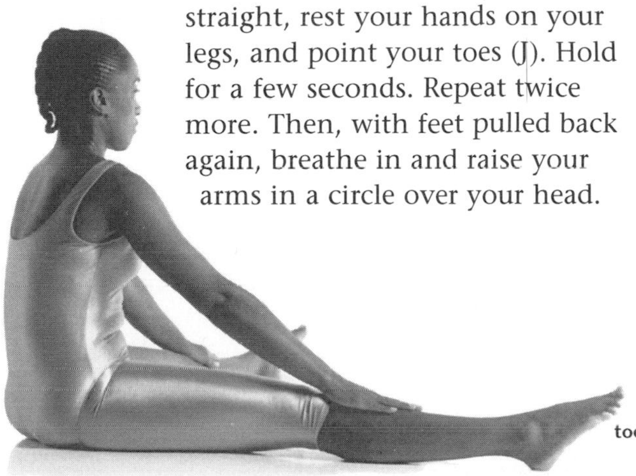

back straight

J

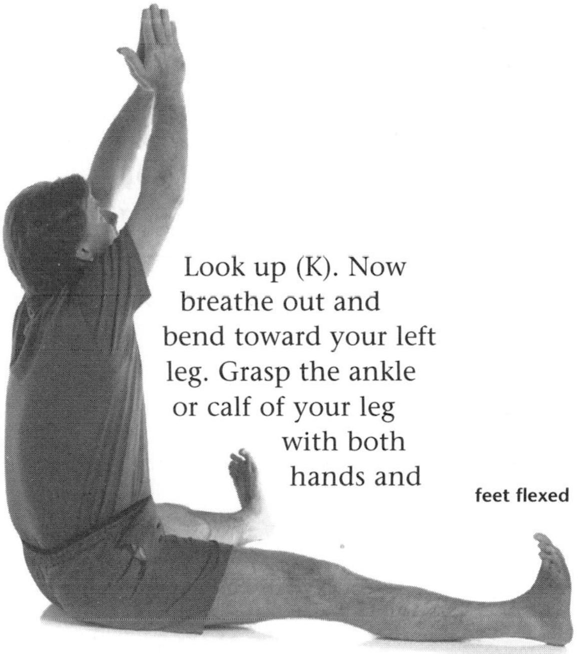

toes pointed

Look up (K). Now breathe out and bend toward your left leg. Grasp the ankle or calf of your leg with both hands and

feet flexed

K

bend your elbows slightly, pulling your upper body *gently* toward your leg (L, next page). Keep your knees straight. (If you can reach your toes comfortably and still bend your arms, wrap your left hand around the big toe (M)

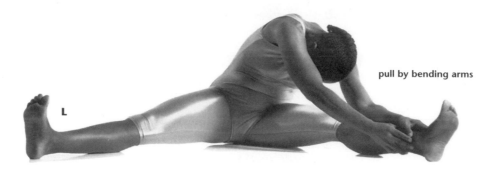

pull by bending arms

L

and grasp the arch of your foot with your right hand.) Your breath should be completely out. Hold for a few seconds, then breathe in, raise your arms in a circular motion overhead, look up, then breathe out and lower your arms in another circle to your sides.

Repetitions: 3 on each side

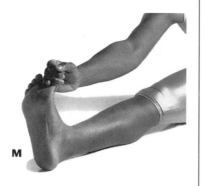

M

Now lean forward toward the center as far as you can comfortably and just rest, breathing normally, for a few seconds (N). Again, if you can reach your toes comfortably, wrap your fingers around your big toes.

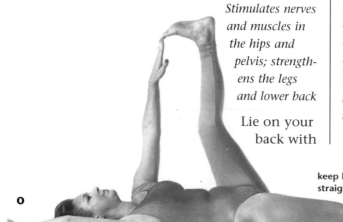

N

Alternate Toe Touch

Stimulates nerves and muscles in the hips and pelvis; strengthens the legs and lower back

Lie on your back with

legs together and arms overhead on the floor. Breathe out completely, then breathe in and raise your left arm and left leg (O). Try to touch your toes without lifting your shoulder off the floor. Breathe out and lower the leg and arm. Repeat with the right leg and arm.

Repetitions: 3 on each side

keep both knees as straight as possible

O

THE REWARDS OF DAILY PRACTICE

Do you remember the story of the Frog Prince? A princess was rewarded for her kindness and constancy to an ugly frog by having the frog turn into a handsome prince! In one of the ancient Yoga books there is a verse that says practice is like poison in the beginning, but like nectar in the end. What this saying means is that at first it can be hard to get started in daily discipline, and the results may seem slow in coming. But if you keep at it, Yoga will become an important part of your day, and you will really miss it if you don't do it. Once established in daily practice, you will begin to feel a steady growth and improvement in yourself; this feeling is very pleasant and will help to make you happy.

Easy Bridge

Improves functioning of thyroid; eases back pain and fatigue; increases circulation to head; helps relieve bedsores

Lying on your back, bend your knees and bring your feet as close to your hips as possible.

Separate your feet several inches. Place your arms, palms down, at your sides. Relax your neck and upper back, breathe out completely, pushing your waist to the floor slightly, then breathe in and raise your hips, arching your back and tucking your chin toward your chest (P). Hold for 1 or 2 seconds, then breathe out and lower. As you become more limber, you can hold on to your ankles for a greater stretch (Q).

Repetitions: 3

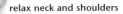

relax neck and shoulders

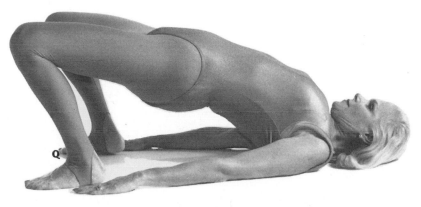

CREATING AN ATMOSPHERE FOR YOGA

The way to build a lasting habit is to make it a ritual. You probably have a set routine that you follow in the morning; you never forget to brush your teeth because by now you do it almost automatically. If you create a routine for daily Yoga practice as well, you will find that eventually your mind will automatically begin turning inward as soon as you put on your exercise clothes or spread out your mat. This is how creating a ritual, by using the same exercise clothes or exercising on the same towel or mat, can help you build a steady daily practice of Yoga.

Corpse Pose

Rests and relaxes entire body

Lie on your back with arms at your sides, palms up. Close your eyes. Let your feet fall apart slightly. Relax your entire body, paying particular attention to your face and stomach. Breathe normally. Rest for at least a minute.

5

RELAXATION AND MEDITATION: 8 MINUTES

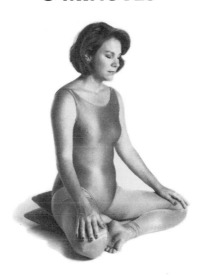

Our world is full of expectations. People want things from us, and we want things for ourselves and others. The constant pull on our attention is often debilitating and fatiguing.

When we're not overloaded with expectations, we're plagued by recriminations. *Why did I do . . . ? What could I have been thinking of when I said . . . ? Who does he think he is to treat me like . . . ?* Scenarios from the past play out in endless loops: *If only . . . I should have . . .*

What effect do these thoughts have on you? Meditation is a way to learn to look more carefully at the many conversations in your mind and gently let them stop. As you observe your thoughts, use the guidelines provided in Chapter 11, in the section "10 Ways to Be Your Own Best Friend," to judge what effect these kinds of thoughts are having on you. Ask yourself what you are doing to yourself with your thoughts: Are you lying to yourself, stealing from yourself, causing harm to yourself?

The meditation segment of your 20-minute workout allows you to draw back from the daily bombardment of wants, needs, and regrets for a few minutes each day and find a resting point where you explore the feeling of *not thinking about anything.* In meditation you will learn to be happy not knowing what comes next, content in the moment, the present. The past and the future—two conditions that dominate probably 90% of our conscious minds—are put on hold for a few minutes. My teacher Lakshmanjoo once said, "The past is dead, the future is not yet born." *In meditation the idea is to concentrate on the present,* only the present. Keep bringing the mind back to the present—and then stop *all* thought. In breaking the cycle of ordinary thought, you get a rest.

As you learn to meditate, try not to expect any particular result. Forget what anybody says about meditation, or what you've read about it elsewhere. *The best experience in meditation comes when you are off guard.* If you don't expect anything, you will never be disappointed, and many times you will be pleasantly surprised. If you have no expectations, you will never get discouraged and stop practicing, and because you don't stop practicing, you will gradually become more and more comfortable in this different and enticing state of meditation. You will look forward to it—like going to meet a good friend or taking a sweet rest.

When you meditate, it appears to the outside world that you are doing "nothing"; actually you are doing something very important for yourself. Our society does not generally approve of the idea of doing "nothing," because it seems unproductive. Americans are trained from childhood that they must give and serve until they die. In Yoga you must learn to give to yourself as well as to others. *In the case of meditation, learning to give to yourself means giving yourself some time each day where you do nothing and think nothing.* You are relaxed and quiet on the outside and relaxed and quiet on the inside. Not planning, not wanting, not remembering, not moving. When you do this successfully you are creating for yourself a new awareness of the powerful creative force that lies within you and supports everything you do. Meditation allows you to reach a source of strength that is always there in you—like fresh water continually refilling a well.

As you begin, you will probably notice your thoughts going off in countless directions. Each time you notice yourself thinking, gently bring your mind back to no thought, without judging. Feeling guilty, frustrated, or self-blaming will not accomplish anything; besides, you want to be a friend to yourself, not punish yourself. *Meditation practice teaches tolerance and patience for yourself.*

HOW CAN I TELL IF I'M PROGRESSING IN MEDITATION?

Progress doesn't have a definition in Yoga, except perhaps the condition that you practice every day. Meditation is such a wide-open experience, so different for every person who practices it, that "progress" cannot be measured. If it could be, progress would become a demand on yourself, and that would be considered unfriendly. If you put yourself in position for meditation experience, without expecting anything, have no doubt that you will achieve the goals you can reasonably expect in meditation—awareness and peaceful silence. "Putting yourself in position" means following the instructions outlined in this chapter: setting aside several undisturbed minutes every day, settling into a position where your body is comfortable and your spine is straight, and then gently withdrawing your mind from thought. This is the only progress you will be looking for.

The Technique

In preparation for meditation, turn off your phone, and be sure no pets are in the room with you. Keep this time for yourself. If you live with small children, meditate while they are sleeping, or ask someone to look after them during your workout.

   During meditation you should not have to have one part of your mind occupied with other concerns. During these 8 minutes, you want all your attention on what you are doing and how you are feeling.

   The best position in which to begin meditation is lying flat on a blanket or large towel, either on the floor or on your bed. Later you can practice a seated position (see Chapter 6), but in the beginning it is important to be as comfortable as possible so that you won't be distracted by a weak back or stiff knees that start to complain after a few minutes of trying to sit upright. Wear socks and cover yourself with a blanket or a shawl or sweater. You'll feel warm after exercising, but during meditation your body temperature will naturally drop slightly as your autonomic nervous system slows your heartbeat and rate of respiration, so guard against becoming chilled. It will be easier to practice if you stay very warm. A covering will also give you a psychological feeling of protection during meditation.

   Your meditation position is designed to keep your spine straight. Don't put a pillow under your head unless you must do so for medical reasons, and then use only a small one. Try not to have any pressure on the back of your neck. If you have a problem with lower back tension, you can put some pillows under your legs—the best place is beneath your thighs—to lift your knees slightly and release some of the pressure on your lower back. Place your arms at your sides, close to your body, with the palms of your hands turned up, and let your fingers curl naturally.

When you feel settled and comfortable, it's time to begin your complete relaxation exercise (see below). In this process, which will take about 2 to 3 minutes, you will focus on each part of your body and relax it. Do this by creating a picture of each part of your body in your mind. Don't move your body, don't tense the muscles, just use your mind: think about each area, then relax it, forget about it, and go on to the next. By directing your attention to the different parts of your body and to the idea of relaxation in your mind, you will more easily be able to rest in stillness during meditation.

COMPLETE RELAXATION PROCEDURE

Forehead To begin, close your eyes, and gently turn your attention toward your face. Think of your forehead, and relax it, smooth it out, as if your fingers could smooth out any tension or lines from the inside of your forehead. Relax your eyebrows, and especially the spot between your eyebrows that often holds furrows of tension. Smooth it out with your mind.

Eyes Keeping your eyes closed, imagine you are looking into a mirror. What color are your eyes? What shape are they? Now imagine you are closing your eyes; the image of yourself in the mirror fades away, but your eyes stay relaxed. Think of the circle of muscles around your eyes and let them go loose, so your eyes rest motionless in the sockets.

Face Extend the feeling of softness and relaxation to the skin of your cheeks. Particularly relax the corners of your mouth. Feel the skin on your face soften and loosen, as if it were made out of warm, pliable wax. Move your attention to your mouth, and relax your lips. Think of your teeth and imagine them loosening in the gums. Relax the roof of your mouth, and let your tongue rest. Let your lower jaw loosen and relax. You can even let your mouth hang open slightly if it feels more comfortable that way.

Neck and Shoulders Gently bring your attention down to your throat and relax your neck muscles. Think of your vocal cords resting. Think about the shape of your collarbone and feel it soften. Bring your attention to your shoulder joints and imagine them opening, so your arms drop toward the floor slightly.

Arms and Hands Now begin to move your attention slowly down your arms, relaxing each section. Let your upper arms relax, then think about your elbows. Focus on the inside of your elbows; how do they feel? Relax them. Then move your mind down your forearms to your wrists. Think of your wrist bones, and the pulse in your wrists, and relax them. Finally, think about your hands—the shape of your fingers, the lines in your palms. Without moving them, let your hands go completely limp, just like a sleeping baby's hands.

Chest and Stomach Gently bring your attention up into your chest. Think about your heart and your lungs, and mentally tell them to

HOW TO ATTAIN A DEEP RELAXATION IN A SHORT TIME

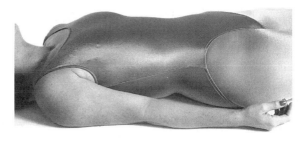

Learn what parts of your body hold tension most, and practice releasing the tension completely. Learn this by observing carefully throughout the day how your body feels when you are at work or at home, moving around or sitting still. Then practice relaxing those parts. This can be done at your desk or in any situation where you have extra time or have an uncomfortable wait, such as in a doctor or dentist's office, in airports or on a plane, or in traffic jams.

For most people, the eyes, jaw, stomach, hands, and feet hold tension most often. You can do a mini relaxation anytime just by concentrating on those particular areas. Notice how they feel, and consciously relax them. Let your eyes droop. Let your mouth fall open and your chin go slack. Shake out your hands and let them fall to your sides. Take a full, complete breath in, then just sigh it out and let your stomach muscles relax. Think of gravity letting go completely.

take a rest for a few minutes. Think about how they look, then take in a deep, complete breath, filling your lungs; then sigh the breath out and relax your heart and lungs at the same time. Let your breath go back to normal. Think of your stomach muscles, and relax them. Relax all your internal organs. Imagine them floating inside your body, at rest.

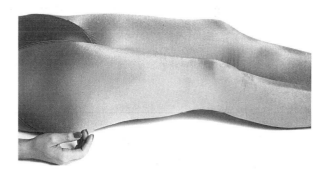

Hips, Legs, and Feet   Think of your hip joints, and imagine them softening, and opening slightly, so your legs drop toward the floor slightly. Then move that same relaxed feeling down your legs, beginning with the long muscles and bones in your thighs. Think about how they look and feel, and let them become still. Relax your

knee joints, your calves, and then think of your ankles. Let the bones in your ankles relax, and the strong tendons at the back of your ankles. Now move to your feet, and think about how they look. Imagine your toes, without moving them. Notice how they feel. Then simply let them go limp, let them fall outward slightly, and relax.

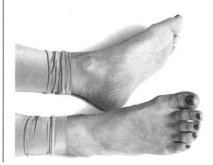

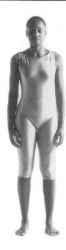

THE TURN

The key to meditation was taught to me by the great Yoga master Lakshmanjoo. One summer in Kashmir he was trying to explain this concept to me. All of a sudden he got up from his seat in the teahouse in his garden where I took my lessons, ran down the steps to the path, and took a soldier's stance, salute and all. He said, "Now, Alice, you are Mrs. Gandhi reviewing the troops. I am the troops. Here we are marching, marching. Soon we come to the end of the parade ground. What do we do? We have to turn around and come back! It's in the turn, Alice, the secret is in the turn!" The turn, the middle point between two breaths, between two steps, between two thoughts, *that* is where the secret to meditation lies. At the turn, you are neither here nor there, neither in nor out, you have no goals, no expectations. It is like a suspension in time, full of possibilities—far beyond ordinary thought.

Spine Now move your attention up the back of your legs to the base of your spine. Think about how your spine looks. Imagine the building blocks of your vertebrae, hollow inside, protecting the spinal cord and all those important nerve connections. Visualize the disks cushioning each vertebra. Your spine is not perfectly straight, but has a slight curve. Imagine your spine as healthy, strong, and relaxed as you move your attention from one part of your back to another. Begin at your lower back. It is slightly elevated from the floor. Relax any tension; let it go. Then move your mind up to the area just in back of your waist; relax it. Relax the spot between your shoulder blades, in your upper back. Then let your neck relax. Notice the spot right at the base of your skull where your spinal cord leads up into your brain. Relax that spot; feel it soften. Then imagine the bones of your skull opening slightly, and your brain simply floating inside. Imagine your brain as a balloon that's been overfilled; mentally let some of the air out, so your brain feels more relaxed, quieter, just resting.

INVITE MEDITATION

Now it's time to go into meditation. Bring your attention gently back to your forehead, and think of the sound "OM" (pronounced "ohm"). This is a *mantram,* a sound that will help to give you a particular feeling of stillness. This *mantram* has been used by practitioners of Yoga for thousands of years to achieve that effect. Say it to yourself a few times, letting the sound resonate inside your head, and thinking only of the sound, nothing else. (If you have my audiocassette program on meditation, I sing this sound to you at the beginning and at the end of your meditation session, as my teacher did with me. Information on the audiocassette can be found in the Appendix, page 140.)

Now begin to look for the feeling of stillness. It is the sensation of not thinking, not reacting, not remembering, not planning, not paying attention to any sounds outside you, but simply resting, observing, attending to the quiet feeling. It is not something that can be drawn out by force. It is always there, but it must be invited, respected, recognized, and enjoyed by your full attention. Don't worry if you can't seem to feel anything except lots of thoughts in the beginning. Just wait, and soon you will begin to notice small moments of silence between the thoughts. Focus on those moments when they are there, and when you notice that thoughts have slipped back in, gently turn your attention away from them into silence again. Concentrate on the space between the thoughts. Don't talk to yourself.

You'll get the best results in meditation if you don't try to force yourself to stop thinking. The mind is a willful child; the more you push against it, the more it will resist. A rigid attitude of forcing your mind to stop thinking is a demand and a form of violence to yourself. Instead, simply continue to gently stop the thoughts as you notice them arising in your mind. Let go of the thoughts without reacting to

them. Observe them as if they were passing by, far in the distance. Tell your mind you will attend to these thoughts later; now you wish to stop thinking. Some people find it helpful to imagine a blank movie screen, or a clear sky, or a calm lake, or some similar mental picture to help in becoming quiet. If this helps you to stop thinking, hold the image in your mind until you feel still, then gently let the image go and keep the feeling.

If you fall asleep, don't worry. This is a stage that many students go through at first. You will eventually stay awake as your mind adjusts to the fact that although your body is sending many of the same signals as in sleep (relaxed muscles, slower breathing, eyes closed, etc.), your mind is being directed to stay attentive. The sleep that you experience in meditation is extremely restful, because you slip into the deepest sleep state; you'll awake very refreshed. If you are worried about sleeping through an appointment, or if you are practicing in the morning and worry about being late for work, allow an extra 10 minutes just in

PRATYAHARA

In Yoga, the word for a beginning experience of preparation for meditation is *pratyahara*, which means "withdrawal of the mind from the senses." The analogy is made to a tortoise, which can withdraw its five limbs (arms, legs, and head) into its shell. Of course, we have more than just five senses. We have a sense of heat and cold, for example, and a sense of balance. Most significantly, we have our kinesthetic sense, the awareness of where our body is in space.

The experience of losing awareness of your hands, or feet, or other parts of your body is related to this loss of the kinesthetic sense. It is a common experience in meditation that is sometimes called "loss of body consciousness." If you feel that sensation, it probably means that you have become very quiet indeed.

case. Or you can learn to wake yourself up by telling yourself, before you start, how long you wish to meditate, just as you can tell yourself, when you go to bed, what time you wish to wake up. At the end of the specified time, you will automatically start to come out of meditation.

COMMON EXPERIENCES IN MEDITATION

From the discussion at the beginning of this chapter, you will have learned that *no* experience is the best experience in meditation! Nevertheless, sensations, images, and other experiences do often occur, and they can be very seductive. When something strange happens in meditation, treat the experience just like any other thought, and gently stop thinking about it.

Many people experience *physical sensations* during the process of relaxation: some examples are feeling weightless or very heavy, feeling that part of the body is twisted, or feeling very hot. Sometimes there is a feeling of pressure in one part of the body, such as the forehead or a place on the spine, or a slight dizziness. Most physical sensations are caused by a block or resistance to the flow of energy throughout the body or a weakness of the nervous system; regular practice of Yoga *asans* will remove the block and strengthen the nervous system.

Mental sensations are also commonly experienced: some examples are seeing lights and colors, or experiencing images and events similar to dreams. Lights and colors are usually manifestations of the electrical activity in your brain; dreamlike images are expressions from the subconscious that take a shape when you are relaxed and off guard, just as in sleep.

AFTER MEDITATION

When your meditation period is over, don't jump right up. Before you move a muscle, take a look at your mind. Ask yourself: *What am I feeling now? Who is feeling this? Where is the feeling coming from?* If you can remember the feeling of meditation, you can reproduce it any time of day that you need or want it.

Start moving now by wiggling your fingers, then your toes. Make a fist and release it. Pull your toes back toward your face. Take a deep breath and stretch your arms and legs. Get up slowly and go about your day refreshed and energized. And it took only 20 minutes!

You can practice the technique of meditation at other times of the day not only by remembering the feeling of meditation but also by constantly reminding ("reminding") yourself to notice what is happening right now. Try to become completely aware of this second. Try to live in the moment.

6

THE 20-MINUTE CHALLENGE

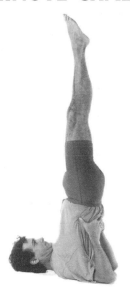

After you've practiced the basic routine for several weeks, you may wish to move on to a more challenging workout. Those of you who have practiced Yoga before will enjoy a more vigorous routine. Remember that Yoga is not competitive, so it really does not matter whether you learn many more complicated exercises or not. The important thing is paying attention to what you *are* doing—whatever the level of difficulty.

Challenge in Yoga is defined not only by physical difficulty but also by mental attention. The effect of Yoga exercise can be described as 10% physical and 90% mental. This means that the results have more to do with the attention and concentration you put into your practices than with the actual physical movements. This is why you can get as much of a challenge with simple exercises as you can with more complicated ones.

Having said that, it is also true that a new routine freshens your attention. When you've done the same routine hundreds of times, you don't have to think so much about what you're doing, and it's easier for your mind to wander. Learning new exercises and varying your routine help prevent boredom and give you a greater repertoire of poses from which you can create your own routines if you wish.

The times for each portion of the workout remain the same, but the emphasis changes. The breathing segment introduces a new breath technique that equalizes the two sides of your body and focuses your attention. The *asan* segment gives your nerves, joints, and muscles a different sort of workout: poses that require a more intense stretch and more strength and stamina.

Notes About Breath

In your breathing exercises now, you should strive for a longer, smoother, deeper breath pattern. In the Complete Breath, time yourself every few days with a watch or clock that has a second hand. Make your inhalation and exhalation equal. Time your most comfortable breath length; if you've been breathing 10 seconds in, 10 seconds out, increase to 12 in, 12 out. Practice this new length for a few weeks before extending it further. Remember that focusing on the sound of the breath increases concentration, reduces outside distractions, and directs your mind toward stillness.

The Alternate Nostril Breath is added both for practice in extending the breath and to make sure that both sides of the nose are open. As you progress in Yoga, unblocked breathing becomes more important. You'll notice a difference in the way *asans* feel and a different effect in meditation when both sides are flowing evenly. (See page 25 for some ways to unblock your breath.) If you practice your workout first thing in the morning, check—before you get out of bed—if one nostril is blocked. To clear it, step out of bed first on the opposite foot. For example, if your left nostril is blocked, put your weight on your right foot first. The blocked side will clear very soon. (This also brings a more subtle effect of balance to your whole day.)

Be sure you've found a seated position for breathing that is so steady you can sit for several minutes without discomfort. If you notice fatigue or pain in your lower back, knees, or ankles, try adding another cushion under your hips. Sometimes just an inch or two of additional height can eliminate any strain on your back. Remember, it isn't necessary to sit on the floor; if you have a back, knee, or hip problem, you can sit on the edge of a chair for breathing and achieve the same results, or even lie on a firm bed or the floor.

Notes About *Asans*

The *asans* in this workout have been chosen to give you a more vigorous routine. (The *asans* included in Chapter 8, "Toning and Shaping with Yoga," are also excellent for a more physically demanding workout. Do the two routines alternately for variety in your daily workout.) These exercises call for greater strength and stamina—especially the new balance poses—and many include several seconds of holding. Whenever you hold a position in Yoga, you increase its effectiveness by allowing more oxygen into the muscles and prolonging the pressure on glands and organs. In a holding position you relax every muscle except the ones you need to use for the exercise. You focus your breath, usually a relaxed breath pattern. At the same time, you improve your concentration by focusing your attention on stillness.

You'll notice a surge in energy after doing a routine like this; it's

THE *ASAN* POINT

Every Yoga *asan* involves three aspects—body, breath, and mind. When you move into position, first make sure your body is in the correct position, including the position of each finger and the focus of your eyes. Use only the muscles you need and relax the rest. For instance, when you do the Dancer Pose, a natural reaction (as in any balance pose) is to tighten the stomach and hold the breath. Many people also tighten their facial muscles as a way of "concentrating" better. Consciously relax your stomach, your breath, and your face.

Next, relax your breath, or, if you're doing a movement exercise, breathe deeply and slowly through your nose. If you're holding a pose, let your breath relax into a natural resting pattern, characterized by a small inhalation, a slightly longer exhalation, and then a pause before you breathe in again. It's similar to your natural breath when you're resting. Try not to manipulate your breath; just let your body decide how to breathe. Focus on the sound of the breath.

The third aspect of the *asan* point is the mind. Stop talking to yourself, just as in meditation. Empty your mind of conversation for the few seconds that you hold the pose. When you do this properly, your entire *asan* routine will give you most of the benefits of meditation.

as if the exercises release energy in you that has been pent-up, locked up in muscle tension and fatigue.

Vigorous *asan* routines replace energy rather than using it up.

Notes About Meditation

In this workout, you may try a seated position for meditation if you wish, and if you have already established a very comfortable seated position for breathing. Remember that the most important aspect of meditation is not the position of your body but the position of your mind. If your body is complaining about its back, or hips, or knees, you will not be able to be silent in your mind. The body is very persistent in letting you know about discomfort of any kind, and it does no good to ignore it—it won't go away for very long. And medita-

tion should never be viewed as a punishment for body or mind, or something you force on yourself. You should enjoy it. So go into a seated meditation only if you are completely comfortable in a seated position for breathing. Otherwise, lie down as before. You may wish to do part of your meditation seated and part lying down at first: begin in a seated position, and then, if you feel your body getting tired, lie down and continue your meditation. You can gradually work up to a longer time in a seated position.

FINDING A COMFORTABLE SEATED POSITION

Take the time to experiment with many different cushions. You'll do best with firmly filled cushions that hold their shape even when you sit on them. Most people need to raise their hips by 3 to 6 inches in order to take the strain off the lower back. When you sit at the right height for you, your pelvis will tilt forward slightly, your back will stay relaxed and straight, and your knees will touch the floor. It helps to sit on the front half of your cushions to give you some help with that tilt. To adjust your position even further, lean forward, arch your back slightly, and then straighten up again.

Keep the cushions you use for Yoga separate. Like your personal mat or blanket, they should be used only for Yoga. When you pick them up, it will increase your mood for practice. Your hands should be relaxed, like a baby's hands. Try placing your hands on your thighs or knees, palms down; this gives some support to your back as well. Or rest your hands in your lap.

Be sure you're warm enough. Even if you're warm from having exercised, throw on a sweater or shawl. Wear socks. Your body temperature will drop just as it does when you're lying down, and chilled muscles get tight faster. Staying warm will enhance your meditation by keeping circulation active.

It can't be stressed enough that comfort is the most important aspect of your seated position. If you're not comfortable, you won't be able to relax or concentrate. Find a comfortable position for meditation and stick with it; do not change it.

BREATHING: 2 MINUTES

Complete Breath

Get into a comfortable position for breathing and begin with 5 to 10 repetitions of the Complete Breath. See Chapter 2, page 28, for a review of this technique.

Alternate Nostril Breath

Balances both sides of body; improves concentration; strengthens respiration

Using your right hand, curl your first and second fingers in toward your palm and hold them with the fleshy part of your thumb. Extend the fourth and fifth fingers straight. Close your right nostril with your thumb and breathe in through your left nostril (A). Breathe completely and slowly, just as in the Complete Breath. Then close your left nostril with the fourth and fifth fingers, and breathe out through your right nostril (B). Breathe in through the right nostril, then close with your thumb and breathe out, then in, through your left nostril. Continue for 5 to 10 breath cycles. Focus on the sound of the breath. Breathe evenly and smoothly.

Repetitions: 5-10

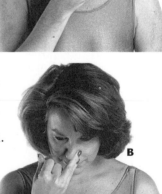

Standing 8-Count Breath

Straighten your legs, make sure joints and muscles are relaxed, then stand up. Close your eyes, balance equally on both feet, and do 3 Complete Breaths, counting 8 on each part of the breath. See page 30 for a review of this technique.

WARM-UPS: 2 MINUTES

Use the same warm-up routine as in the regular workout (see Chapter 3, page 31).

ASANS: 8 MINUTES

Standing Sun Pose (pictured, p. 44)

With feet parallel, breathe out, then breathe in as you raise your arms in a wide circle overhead and bring your palms together. Look up. Then breathe out and bend forward, tuck your head, grasp your ankles or calves, bend your elbows and gently pull your upper body toward your legs without bending your knees. Hold for a few seconds, then breathe in and straighten, lifting your arms in a circle overhead. Look up, then breathe out and lower your arms.

Repetitions: 3

Dancer Pose and Variation

Strengthens the lower back; limbers and strengthens the hips and thighs; improves mental poise, posture, balance, and concentration; strengthens ankles; relieves upper back tension

From a standing rest position, bend your right leg and grasp your right foot with your left hand (C). Throughout the exercise, steady yourself by fixing your gaze on one spot on the wall in front of you. Check to be sure your stomach muscles are relaxed and your breathing steady. Slowly move into the completed Dancer Pose by raising your right arm straight up toward the ceiling so it is next to your ear and pulling your right leg *up* and *back* as far as possible without strain (D). Check to be sure your supporting leg is straight. Relax your stomach, breathe normally, and keep your gaze fixed on one spot. Hold for 10 to 15 seconds.

Repetitions: 1 on each side

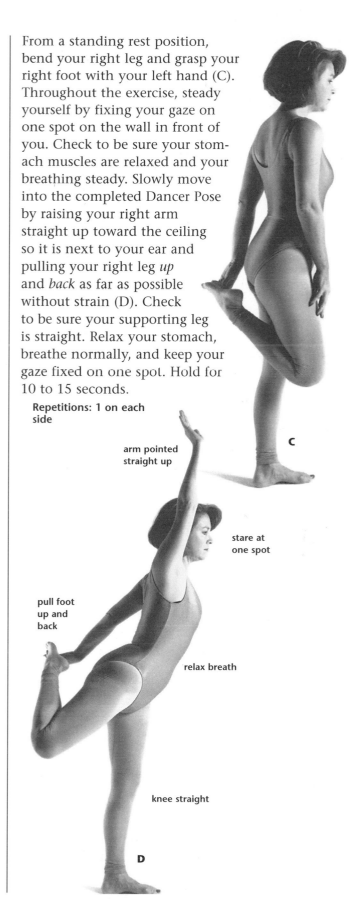

arm pointed straight up

stare at one spot

pull foot up and back

relax breath

knee straight

C

D

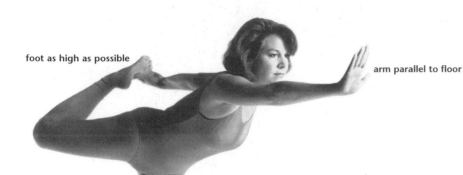

foot as high as possible

arm parallel to floor

knee straight

E

Maintaining your gaze and still breathing normally, slowly lower your body into the extended position (E). *In addition to the benefits of the Dancer Pose, this variation stretches the back of the legs and increases strength and stamina.* Keep your right leg as far up and back as possible. Your right arm extends straight ahead. Your left (supporting) leg remains straight. Hold for 5 to 10 seconds. Stare at one spot for balance. Don't strain. Come back to a standing rest position, and switch sides.

Repetitions: 1 on each side

Eagle Pose

Improves concentration and balance; strengthens nervous system

Stare at one spot on the floor for balance while you get into this exercise. Bend your left leg slightly and wrap your right leg over and behind it (if you can't reach behind the leg, just go as far as you can). When you're steady, bend your torso and place your *left* elbow on your *right* knee. Then place your right elbow *inside* your left elbow, turn your hands toward each other, and clasp your fingers. Bend your head so your forehead rests on your hands (F). Hold for a few seconds, breathing normally. Slowly untwist and switch sides.

Repetitions: 1 on each side

supporting knee bent

F

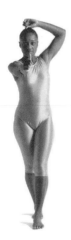

ARJUNA THE ARCHER

Arjuna is a central character in a long Indian epic called *The Mahabharata*. He was a prince of the warrior class. A story is told of when he was studying the art of archery. He and his classmates were told to draw their bows and aim for a bird sitting in a distant tree. As they held the position, their teacher asked each student in turn what he saw. The first answered, "A field, some trees, and one tree that has a bird in it." Another answered, "I see only the tree with the bird in it." When it came Arjuna's turn, he answered, "I see only the eye of the bird." This story illustrates the powers of concentration required of a master, and that they may be realized by practicing *asans* such as the Archer Pose.

Archer Pose

Increases mental poise and one-pointedness; may help heal addiction

The ideal position for your feet in this pose is pointed straight ahead, one directly in front of the other. Until you master the exercise, you may keep your feet slightly apart for balance. Start with the *left* foot forward and the *right* foot back. Extend your right arm straight ahead and position the hand as if you were holding a bow, with the thumb pointed up. Place your left hand on your head with fingers curled to hold the string of the bow (G). Breathe in, looking forward at your right thumb, then slowly and carefully breathe out and turn toward the right, keeping your right arm outstretched and following your thumb with your gaze (H). Twist back as far as you can, hold a few seconds, breathing gently, then inhale as you twist slowly back to face front. Relax your arms and switch positions (left hand outstretched, right hand on your head) but keep your feet in the same position. Stare at the thumb of your outstretched hand. Breathe in, then slowly and carefully twist back to the left this time (I). Hold for a few seconds, breathing gently, then breathe in and return to the front. Relax your arms. Change the position of your feet so the right foot is forward and repeat both movements.

Repetitions: 1 on each side

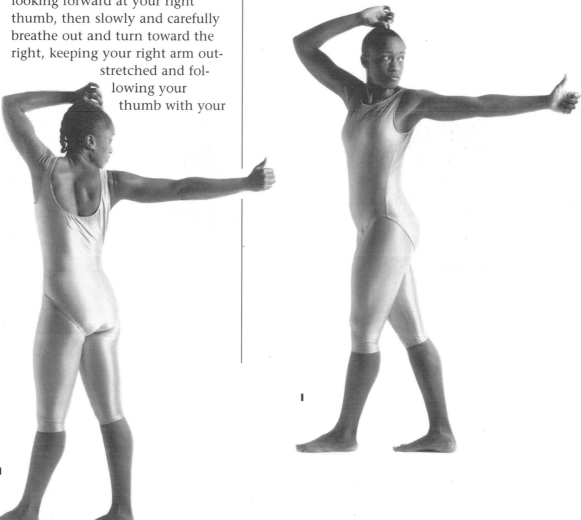

G

H

I

Baby Pose *(pictured, p. 46)*

Sit on your feet, bend forward, and rest your head on the floor. Bend your elbows so they rest on the floor. Relax completely, breathing gently, for at least 1 minute.

Front Crow

Strengthens arms and upper back; improves blood flow throughout internal organs and spine

Squat on your toes and place your hands on the floor between your knees, about a foot apart. Bend your elbows and place the inside of your knees against your elbows (J). Holding that position, carefully lean forward, resting your bent legs on the back of your elbows, until your feet come off the floor (K). Don't hold your breath; let your body decide how to breathe. Hold the position for at least 5 seconds if you can.

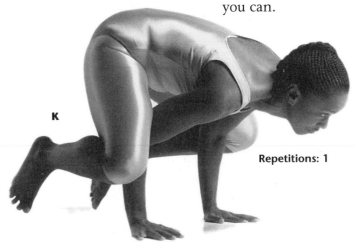

Repetitions: 1

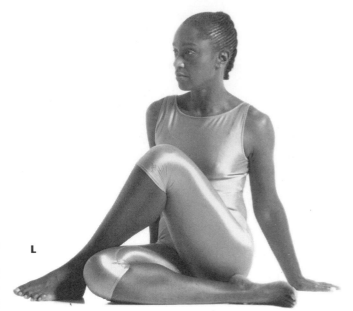

foot close to hip

Spine Twist

Improves digestion; limbers and tones entire spine; strengthens and limbers rib cage; relieves chronic constipation; helps relieve bladder, urinary tract, and prostate problems

Sit with legs outstretched. Bend both knees. Rest your right leg on the floor, and lift your left leg over the right knee; the left foot should be flat (L). Sit up very straight, reach your right arm across your left knee, push the knee as far right as it will go, and grasp the right knee with your right hand; this locks the lower back into position. Your right arm is on the *outside* of your raised (left) leg. Now place your left arm behind you, straighten it, and point the fingers in toward the base of your spine. Look forward, breathe in, then breathe out and twist toward the left as far as possible (M). Look far to the left and stare at one spot. Hold for several seconds, breathing

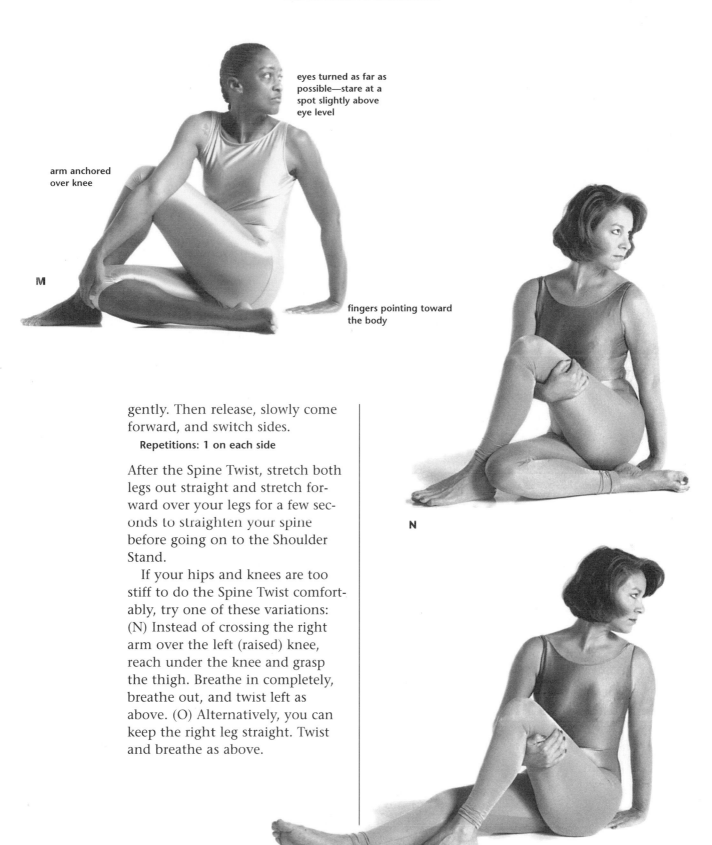

eyes turned as far as possible—stare at a spot slightly above eye level

arm anchored over knee

M

fingers pointing toward the body

N

O

gently. Then release, slowly come forward, and switch sides.

Repetitions: 1 on each side

After the Spine Twist, stretch both legs out straight and stretch forward over your legs for a few seconds to straighten your spine before going on to the Shoulder Stand.

If your hips and knees are too stiff to do the Spine Twist comfortably, try one of these variations: (N) Instead of crossing the right arm over the left (raised) knee, reach under the knee and grasp the thigh. Breathe in completely, breathe out, and twist left as above. (O) Alternatively, you can keep the right leg straight. Twist and breathe as above.

Shoulder Stand

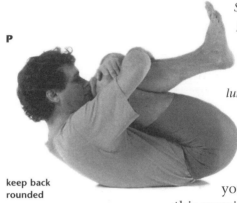

keep back
rounded

*Stimulates thyroid and
parathyroid; enhances
function of all vital
organs; relieves ten-
sion on heart and
lungs; relaxes nervous
system; removes
fatigue*

If you have a
disk problem in
your neck, do not do
this exercise or the Plow.
Substitute the Easy Bridge (pictured on page 49) instead. This
exercise has many benefits. Hold it
as long as you can comfortably.
Start by sitting with knees drawn
up to chest and arms wrapped
around knees. Gently roll back
and forth a few times to make sure
that the spine is in place with no
pinched nerves or strained muscles
(P). Then roll all the way back,
keeping knees to forehead, and
immediately support your back
with your hands (Q). Hold this
position until you feel
steady, then slowly
straighten your legs
(R). If your legs
appear to be more at

support back
with hands

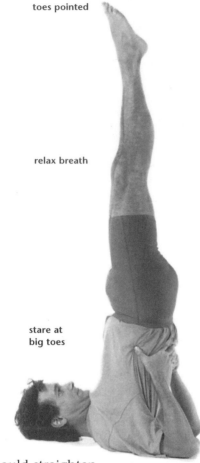

toes pointed

relax breath

stare at
big toes

R

45° angle, move
your hands down
your back
toward the floor
and tuck your
chin into your
chest; your legs should straighten
a bit more. Fix your gaze on the
space between your big toes. Relax
your breath. Hold as long as you
can comfortably.

Go on to the Plow or come out
of the pose by bending your knees
and bringing them to your forehead. Slowly roll forward, rounding your back, until you come all
the way up to a seated position.
Bend forward for a few seconds to
be sure the blood doesn't drain
from your head too fast.

Repetitions: 1

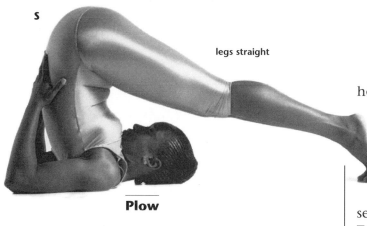

legs straight

Plow

Stimulates thyroid; stretches entire spine; reduces body fat; stretches arteries and veins

Do not do this exercise if you have a disk problem in your neck. From the Shoulder Stand, bend your knees until they touch your fore-head, then slowly straighten your legs over your head until your toes touch the floor (S). If this is comfortable, you can straighten your arms and place your hands, palms down, on the floor. Hold for several seconds. Relax your breath. To come out of the pose, bend your knees and bring them back to your forehead. Slowly roll forward to a seated position and bend your head forward for a few seconds.

Repetitions: 1

Bow Pose

Relieves chronic constipation; improves functioning of digestive system; strengthens back and thigh muscles; increases vitality

Lie on your stomach with your forehead on the floor and your knees bent.

Reach back and grasp your ankles (T). Breathe out completely, then breathe in and lift up, balancing on your stomach (U). Look up. Breathe out and lower to the starting position.

Repetitions: 3

Turn on your back and rest in the Corpse Pose (page 50) for several seconds before meditation.

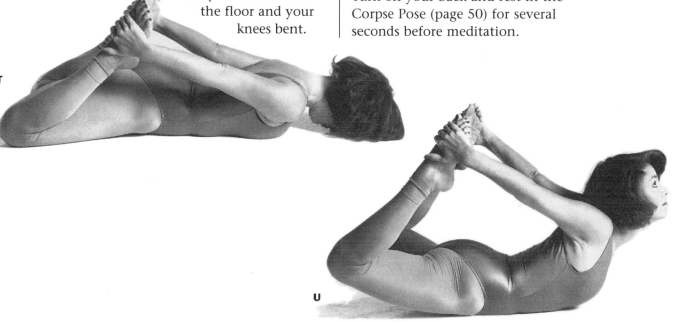

Meditation

Take your most comfortable position, either seated or lying down, for meditation. For a review of the relaxation and meditation procedure, see Chapter 5. Relaxing in a seated position is similar to lying down; the trickiest part will be to keep your back straight without tensing it. Over time, you will learn how to hold just the postural muscles in your back steady and relax the other back muscles so you feel relaxed but don't slouch forward. Hold your head so it balances straight on your neck; avoid bending your head forward or back. Go through your relaxation procedure from your forehead to your toes and back up, just as you do lying down. Keep your body warm.

7

YOGA AND WOMEN'S ISSUES

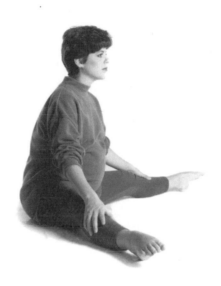

Yoga and Change

Every month women's bodies go through a radical change in preparation for possible pregnancy. As the hormones shift their delicate balance, these changes are experienced as physical and emotional feelings. For some, these monthly changes bring several days of discomfort and stress; for others, it is a minor inconvenience. But no woman can ignore this regular change in her body and mind.

Other enormous changes occur at menopause, sometime around age 50, when a woman's reproductive system slows down and eventually stops. Some women sail right through these years with little or no discomfort, while others seem to get bogged down in uncomfortable and often unwelcome sensations as their body adjusts to a new chemical balance.

Living with such hormonal changes on a regular basis probably makes any type of change easier to handle. Change is inevitable in the world, so it makes sense to make it work *for* you instead of resisting it. In Yoga, being able to accept change and move on is a central concept, primarily because resisting change takes so much energy. Why waste your energy on something that will only hold you back? In Yoga we often use the metaphor of water to describe the ideal stance in moving through a turbulent world. If you make yourself like water, every action will be easier. Yoga helps you to be fluid in change. It is said that Yogis love water because it has no resistance. Yet that doesn't mean water is not powerful; water, over time, can carve out deep canyons and wear down the hardest rock. In the same way, if you learn to welcome change, you will gain great strength and happiness.

Yoga is ideally suited for helping you adjust to change—hormonal or otherwise. By reinforcing positive change through relaxation, steadiness, flexibility, and other qualities, Yoga helps you enjoy the many inevitable changes that occur at different times in your life. In this chapter are three 20-minute workouts designed for PMS, pregnancy and after birth, and menopause.

Premenstrual Syndrome (PMS)

In the United States and Britain it's sometimes called "the Curse" or given a name like "Charlie" or "George." In Jamaica and Nigeria it's called "Flowers." In some other parts of the world, the words for it mean "being unwell." Every culture has its slang and myths about menstruation and its associated symptoms, including the constellation of symptoms that we call PMS, or premenstrual syndrome. PMS affects about half of all women in one way or another, with any combination of the following symptoms:

Physical Water retention; weight gain; swelling of feet, ankles, or hands; tender breasts; headache; fatigue; constipation; food cravings; skin eruptions.

Emotional Anxiety; depression; irritability; forgetfulness; inability to concentrate; tension; mood swings; feeling out of control and fearful.

Of course, many of these symptoms happen at other times of the month. Talk with your physician, and keep a record of symptoms to discover any patterns in their occurrence.

HOW YOGA CAN HELP

Yoga practice will teach you how to observe your reactions and manage stress, relax tension in your muscles, and become more centered and aware. The exercises included in the 20-minute workout variation for PMS are gentle stretches that release muscle tension, ease lower back stiffness, regulate breathing, and improve circulation. Breathing, relaxation, and meditation techniques are very important during this time to build concentration and strength. Irritability, depression, and moodiness can be greatly eased by regular meditation, which will help to stabilize your emotions. Use this time to observe your reactions and feelings and learn to be happy with who you are. Set some time aside each day to learn to be happy alone.

We recommend that you *not* practice strenuous Yoga exercises during the days when menstrual flow is heaviest—it could result in hemorrhage or extreme nervous upset. During those days, using the routine that follows, eliminate the Knee Swings and Alternate Toe Touch, and give the extra time to relaxation and meditation.

The 20-Minute PMS Workout

BREATHING: 2 MINUTES

Arched Breath *(pictured, p. 27)*

In a kneeling position, or any comfortable seated position, breathe in as you arch forward, breathe out as you round backward.

Repetitions: 3

Complete Breath *(full description, pp. 28–29)*

In a comfortable seated position, breathe in from the belly up, breathe out from the chest down.

Repetitions: 5-10

Standing 8-Count Breath *(full description, p. 30)*

Straighten your legs, massaging knees and ankles if necessary. Then stand up and continue breathing evenly to a count of 8 (or begin with 5).

Repetitions: 3

WARM-UPS: 2 MINUTES

Follow the same routine as in the regular workout, but eliminate the Side Stretch (you'll do it as part of the *asan* segment instead).

ASANS: 8 MINUTES

Arm Stretch

Stimulates the endocrine system; improves upper-body circulation; stretches the muscles of the rib cage; gradually tightens the skin on the back of the upper arm

Standing with feet parallel, bring your arms straight out in front at shoulder height, palms together (A).

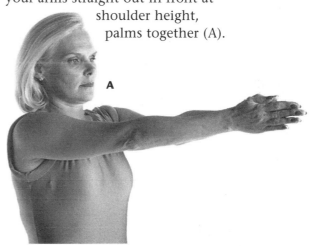

A

Breathe out. Breathe in as you slowly move your arms to the back, keeping them as high as possible and turning the palms toward the outside by rotating inward (B). Hold a second or two, then breathe out and return to the front position.

Repetitions: 5-10

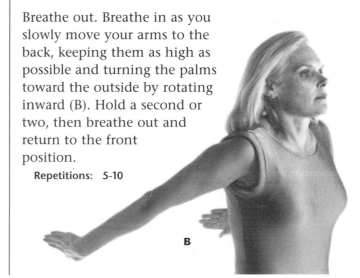

B

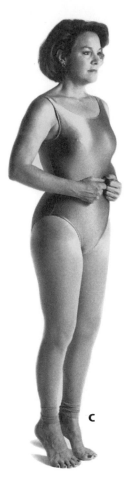

Easy Balance

Improves respiration; oxygenates blood; strengthens ankles and calves; improves balance

Breathe out, arms at your sides. Staring at one spot to help maintain balance, breathe in completely, stretch up on your toes, and press your fists into your diaphragm (C). (Be sure you are not pressing into your rib cage, but directly below it.) Breathe out and relax, lowering your arms and heels.

Repetitions: 3

Side Stretch (pictured, p. 36)

With legs separated as far as is comfortable and toes pointed forward, breathe in and raise your arms straight out to the sides horizontally. Breathe out and stretch to the left, supporting yourself with your left hand on your left leg, and reaching your right arm straight over your head and eventually parallel to the floor. Keep the body in a plane and look straight ahead. Breathe in and return to the first position, arms outstretched. Breathe out and repeat to the right side.

Repetitions: 3 on each side

Cat Breath

Limbers lower and midback; tightens stomach muscles; improves breathing

Start on hands and knees. Breathe in, arch your back, and look up, so you feel the stretch all along your spine, from tailbone to neck (D). Then breathe out, round your back, and pull in your stomach to increase the forward stretch (E). Tuck your head.

Repetitions: 3

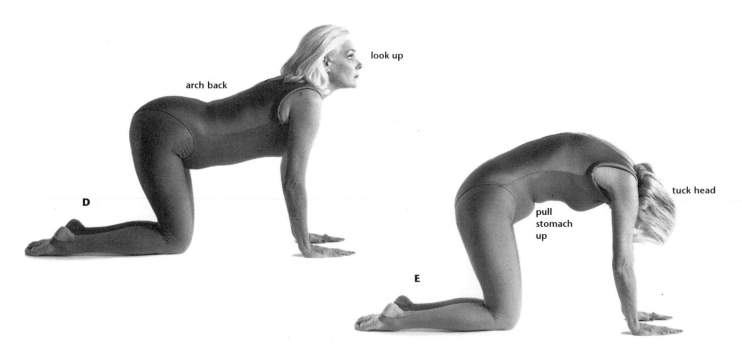

look up

arch back

tuck head

pull stomach up

Lion

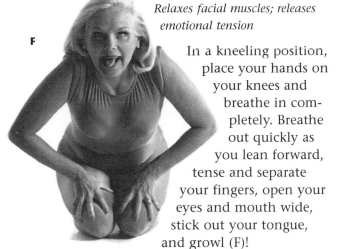

F

Relaxes facial muscles; releases emotional tension

In a kneeling position, place your hands on your knees and breathe in completely. Breathe out quickly as you lean forward, tense and separate your fingers, open your eyes and mouth wide, stick out your tongue, and growl (F)!

Repetitions: 3

Tortoise Stretch *(pictured, p. 47)*

Separate your legs as far as you can comfortably. Lean back on your hands, pull your feet back toward your face, and lift your hips slightly as you push your pelvis forward. Release, point your toes, and sit up for a few seconds with your hands on your thighs. Repeat. Then sit straight with feet pulled back, breathe in, and lift your arms overhead. Look up and stretch. Breathe out and bend toward your left leg. Grasp the leg (or toe, gripped as pictured on page 48)

with both hands and pull gently by bending your arms. Hold for a second or two, then breathe in and bring the arms back up overhead. Look up, then breathe out and repeat on the right side.

Repetitions: 3 on each side

End the Tortoise Stretch by grasping the ankles or toes of both feet and gently holding the forward stretch for a few seconds.

Alternate Toe Touch

(pictured, p. 48)

Lie on your back with arms overhead on the floor. Breathe in and raise the left arm and left leg; try to touch your toes without bending your knee or lifting your shoulder off the floor. Breathe out and lower the leg. Repeat on the opposite side.

Repetitions: 3 on each side

Side Leg Lift

Limbers hips; strengthens lower back, legs, and stomach

Lie on your side, supporting yourself on one arm (G). Breathe out completely. Breathe in and raise

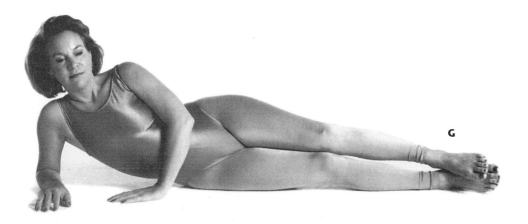

G

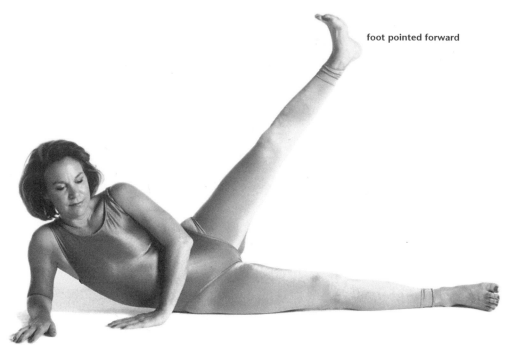

foot pointed forward

H

the top leg straight up, as high as possible without strain (H). Breathe out and lower.

Repetitions: 3 on each side

Walk

Removes fat from hips and thighs; improves circulation in pelvic area and legs

Lying on your back, lift your legs straight up, toes pulled back toward your face, and "walk" your legs back and forth in small steps, keeping your knees straight (I). Continue for as long as you can comfortably. Breathe normally.

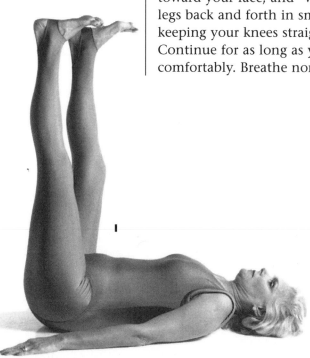

I

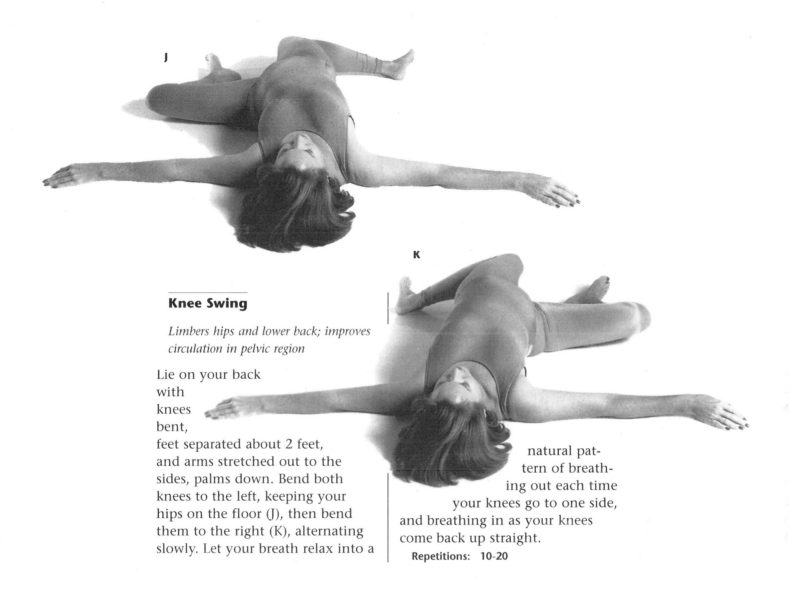

Knee Swing

Limbers hips and lower back; improves circulation in pelvic region

Lie on your back with knees bent, feet separated about 2 feet, and arms stretched out to the sides, palms down. Bend both knees to the left, keeping your hips on the floor (J), then bend them to the right (K), alternating slowly. Let your breath relax into a natural pattern of breathing out each time your knees go to one side, and breathing in as your knees come back up straight.

Repetitions: 10-20

Pregnancy

During pregnancy it is not wise to do strenuous Yoga *asans* because the chemical changes in the body caused by Yoga may overstimulate your developing baby. However, after the first trimester, if you have your doctor's permission, you can follow a modified 20-minute workout that will have many beneficial effects for you and your baby. During pregnancy you may do several exercises that release tension in the back and neck and that stretch the hip joints and groin muscles. The main focus of your 20-minute workout during pregnancy should be relaxation and meditation; in this workout meditation is given 12 to 15 minutes. Regular practice of meditation makes for a serene, confident, and relaxed mother and a happy, well-adjusted baby. As you continue to practice your modified 20-minute workout throughout pregnancy, you will build the habit of taking some time for yourself daily, which will help protect you from depression and fatigue when your baby arrives and the new demands start to build. Many mothers who practice Yoga comment that the training in breath techniques helps them have an easier labor and delivery.

BREATHING: 2 MINUTES

Any comfortable seated position for breathing is fine. If you can sit cross-legged comfortably (A), with appropriate support beneath your hips, this position will also help to loosen your hips and relax the muscles you will use in labor and delivery. Practice sitting cross-legged at other times of the day, to loosen the joints even faster.

You can also straddle a pile of cushions or even do breathing exercises lying down with pillows under your thighs (B). This lying-down position is excellent for meditation.

Arched Breath (pictured, p. 27)

In a comfortable seated position, breathe in and arch your back forward, looking up. Breathe out and round your back, tucking your head.

Repetitions: 3

Complete Breath (for review of Complete Breath procedure, see pp. 28–29)

In a comfortable seated position, breathe in and out evenly and smoothly, using the muscles of your diaphragm, rib cage, and chest. Concentrate on the sound of the breath and breathe through your nose.

Repetitions: 5-10

WARMING UP: 1 MINUTE

Shoulder Roll (pictured, p. 34)

Keeping your arms and hands loose at your sides, slowly rotate your shoulders first forward, then backward, several times in each direction.

Repetitions: 3-4 in each direction

A

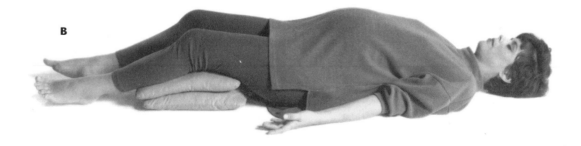

B

Head Roll *(pictured, p. 35)*

Bend your head forward and slowly roll it around to the left, then backward, then to the right, then forward again. Breathe normally. Do not do this exercise if you have a disk problem in your neck.

Repetitions: 3 in each direction

Arm Roll *(pictured, p. 35)*

Stretch arms out to the sides, palms facing outward. Slowly rotate your arms in large circles, then in smaller circles.

Repetitions: 3-5 in each direction

Elbow Twist *(pictured, p. 36)*

Hold arms in front, elbows bent and one hand on top of the other. Breathe in looking forward, then breathe out and twist to one side. Breathe in and return to facing forward.

Repetitions: 3 in each direction

Elbow Touch

Limbers and releases tension in upper back and shoulders; improves breathing

Bring fingertips to shoulders. Breathe out and touch elbows together in front. Breathe in and stretch elbows back as far as possible, keeping arms horizontal.

Repetitions: 3

ASANS: 3 MINUTES

Leg Lift

Strengthens and limbers hip joints; improves circulation in legs

Holding on to a sturdy chair with one or both hands, breathe in and lift your left leg forward, keeping both knees straight and keeping the foot flexed. Breathe out and lower the leg. Repeat to the side and to the back (C).

Repetitions: 3 in each direction with each leg

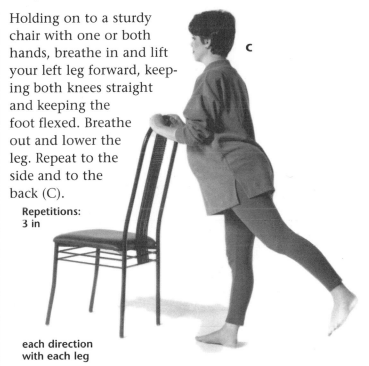

Diamond Pose

Limbers lower back, hips, and groin muscles

Seated, with the soles of your feet together, grasp your ankles with both hands and let your arms rest above your thighs. Breathe in, then breathe out and lean forward, pressing down gently on your thighs with your arms (D). Release.

Repetitions: 3

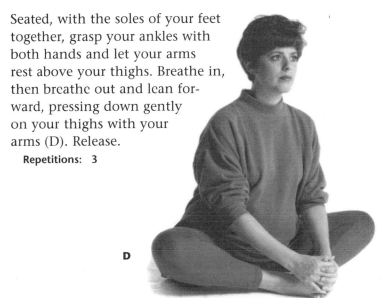

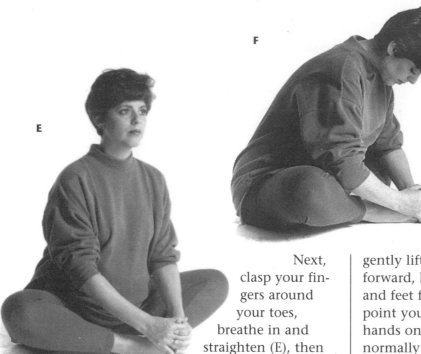

Next, clasp your fingers around your toes, breathe in and straighten (E), then breathe out and bend forward slightly, stretching the hip joints and groin muscles (F).

Repetitions: 3

gently lift your hips, and stretch forward, keeping your heels down and feet flexed (G). Then sit up, point your toes, and rest your hands on your legs (H). Breathe normally throughout.

Repetitions: 2-3

Tortoise Stretch

With legs separated as far as possible, lean back on your hands,

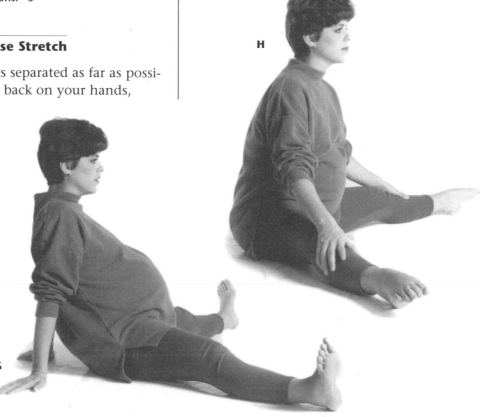

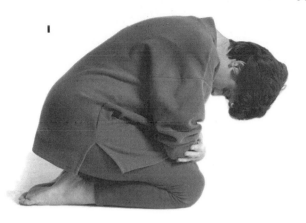

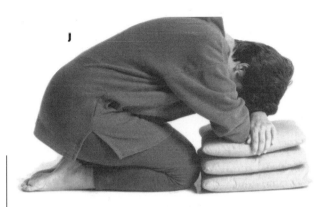

Baby Pose (variations)

In a kneeling position, sitting on your feet, fold your arms on your knees and rest your head forward, in a slightly bent position (I). Alternatively, pile a few cushions in front of your knees and rest your head and folded arms on the pillows (J).

RELAXATION AND MEDITATION: 14 MINUTES

The best position for meditation is lying down, so there is less tension on your lower back. Place a few pillows under your thighs to release back tension.

After the Baby Arrives

During lactation, your body chemistry is radically different, your body is adjusting to a new function, and you need rest above all. Spend most of your 20 minutes on relaxation and meditation; the strength and stability that meditation gives you will be reflected in a happier family and an easier adjustment to a new schedule. As soon as your baby is weaned, you can resume a normal workout routine.

If you wish to do a few exercises while you are nursing, practice the following short routine:

Complete Breath (full description, pp. 28–29)

In a comfortable seated position, breathe in and out evenly and smoothly, using the muscles of your diaphragm, rib cage, and chest. Concentrate on the sound of the breath and breathe through your nose.

Repetitions: 5-10 or more

Arm Roll (pictured, p. 35)

Stretch your arms to the sides, palms facing outward. Slowly rotate your arms in large circles and then smaller circles.

Repetitions: 3-5 in each direction

Head Roll *(pictured, p. 35)*

With arms at your sides or hands on your hips, bend your neck forward toward your chest. Slowly rotate your head in a circle several times in each direction. If you have a disk problem in your neck, do not rotate your head; instead, with your doctor's approval, do simple up-and-down and side-to-side movements.

Repetitions: 3 in each direction

Tree Pose *(pictured, p. 45)*

Standing next to a sturdy chair or wall for support, lift one leg and place the foot on your opposite thigh as high as possible. Steady yourself by staring at one spot for balance. Relax your breath. Slowly lift your arms over your head if you can, or just balance, holding on to your support, for several seconds. Repeat with the other leg.

Keep your hips and knees limber by sitting cross-legged as often as you can.

Repetitions: 1 on each side

Menopause

Why do many women cringe at the thought of "the Big Change," as menopause is often referred to? Is it because it is a marker of growing older (which, sadly, is so looked down upon in our society)? Is it because it is such a permanent signal, marking the end of our reproductive years and the beginning of who-knows-what? I think it is partly because no one teaches us how to navigate this particular passage of life. No one teaches us how to change *happily.* Our mothers spoke in hushed, somber, inhibited tones about "female complaints" and "that age." We grew up dreading an inevitable, mysterious process that would take over our bodies and minds one day and deliver them back to us changed forever, irrevocably, with no recourse. But no one could or would tell us exactly what we would be like afterward. There is very little training to prepare us for aging.

To make things even more complicated, often this is a time when other aspects of our lives are changing as well. Children leave home, careers change direction, interests diverge. Menopause *does* signal a turning point, but it need not be frightening or uncomfortable. It is up to us how we view it, and what we do about it.

Yoga can directly alleviate or reduce many of the most troublesome symptoms of menopause, such as hot flashes, night sweats, vaginal dryness, insomnia, depression, and irritability. Although all Yoga exercises affect the body's chemistry to some extent, there are some exercises that specifically stimulate the glandular and reproductive systems, resulting in a more balanced adjustment of the body's chemistry. The gentle weight-bearing exercises in the routine will help to strengthen bones. Yoga also improves circulation, helps to balance metabolism, and builds a steadiness of mind that evens out many of the emotional ups and downs that many women experience.

Some people think they are too old to change, but change is

always possible, and the rewards of being flexible to change are peace of mind and an openness to new experiences. There is a widespread misconception that Yoga is meant primarily for the young. But in the ancient tradition, some men and women did not start to really practice Yoga until after age 53. It was recognized that until that time, one's attention was naturally focused on one's family and career, and that in the mid-50s, when the children were grown and gone and the business turned over to someone else, one could turn one's attention toward the pursuit of self-awareness and meaning in life.

Of course, not many people practice Yoga these days with the primary goal of self-awareness. But the middle years of life are still a very good time to begin or to resume the study of Yoga. Many women remember a youthful idealism and an openness to self-

knowledge and self-improvement that brought clarity and purpose into their lives. Now is the time to reclaim that attitude and, instead of cursing change for its upheaval, to embrace it for its possibilities and new freedoms.

A woman who is healthy and fit, who knows how to relax, who eats a good, balanced diet, and who is happy with her life will probably not find the symptoms of menopause to be incapacitating. The 20-minute workout described below is designed to help you become that healthy, fit, happy, relaxed person. Exercise raises endorphin levels in your brain (endorphins are the hormones that create feelings of pleasure and relaxation), protects against osteoporosis by strengthening bones, wards off depression, and eliminates anxiety by relaxing body and mind.

20-Minute Workout Variation for Menopause

BREATHING: 2 MINUTES

Complete Breath (full description, pp. 28–29)

In a comfortable seated position, breathe evenly in and out, breathing in from the belly up to the chest and breathing out from the chest to the belly.

Repetitions: 5-10

Alternate Nostril Breath

(pictured, p. 62)

(If one side of your nose is flowing more freely than the other, see discussion of ways to correct this on page 25). In a comfortable seated position, curl the first and second fingers of your right hand inward, close your right nostril with your thumb, and breathe in through the left nostril only. Close the left nostril with your third and fourth fingers, open the right, and breathe out, then in again, through the right nostril. Continue alternating by breathing out, then in, through one side at a time.

Repetitions: 5-10

Standing Reach

Stimulates lymphatic system; strengthens and limbers shoulders and upper back

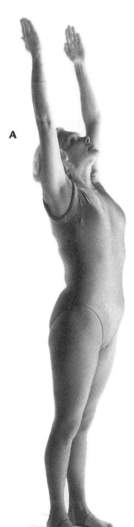

A

Stand with arms at your sides. Breathe out completely. Then start to breathe in as you lift your arms up to the sides and overhead, stretching up as far as you can reach and looking toward the ceiling (A). Then breathe out and bring your arms slowly out to the sides and down again.

Repetitions: 3

WARMING UP: 2 MINUTES

Shoulder Roll (pictured, p. 34)

Keeping your arms and hands loose at your sides, slowly rotate your shoulders first forward, then backward, several times in each direction.

Repetitions: 4-5 in each direction

Throat Stretch

Keeps neck muscles strong and limber; helps to improve circulation to the brain

With lips and teeth together, breathing normally, jut your chin forward, gently tensing the muscles under your chin (B), then retract your head to normal position, and relax your neck. Then turn your head toward the right and repeat: jut your chin forward, gently pushing without straining your neck. You'll feel a slight pull, but be careful not to go too far. Then retract, relax, and come back to the center position. Repeat the stretch, then turn toward the left and repeat.

Repetitions: 3 front, 3 left, and 3 right, alternating

B

Swing Stretch

Improves circulation; limbers the back and legs

Standing with feet slightly separated and arms at sides, breathe in and stretch your arms forward and up as far as you can as in the Standing Reach, then breathe out, bend your knees, and swing your

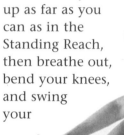

C

arms down in front (C) and all the way back (D). Breathe in and swing back up with arms overhead, straightening your knees. Move with the breath. Stretch up as far as possible each time.

Repetitions: 3

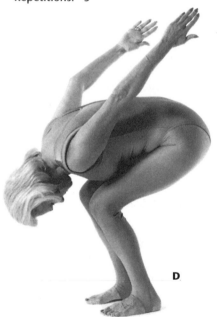

D

Arm Stretch (pictured, p. 73)

Standing with feet slightly apart, lift your arms so they are pointing straight ahead. Breathe out completely. Breathe in and bring your arms straight back as far as you can, squeezing your shoulder blades together and rotating the palms outward. Breathe out and bring your arms back to the front, palms together. Keep elbows straight and arms horizontal throughout.

Repetitions: 5-10

Hip Rock and Rotation

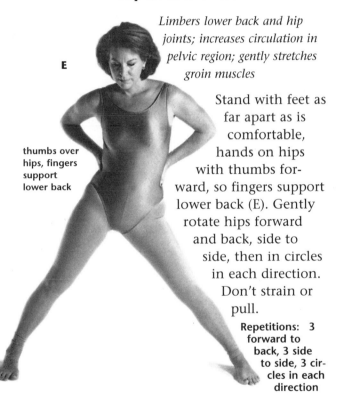

E

thumbs over hips, fingers support lower back

Limbers lower back and hip joints; increases circulation in pelvic region; gently stretches groin muscles

Stand with feet as far apart as is comfortable, hands on hips with thumbs forward, so fingers support lower back (E). Gently rotate hips forward and back, side to side, then in circles in each direction. Don't strain or pull.

Repetitions: 3 forward to back, 3 side to side, 3 circles in each direction

Side Stretch *(pictured, p. 36)*

Stand with feet separated as far as you can comfortably. Breathe in and lift your arms parallel to the floor, then breathe out and bend to the left leg, supporting yourself with your left hand and bringing your right arm straight up and over your head. Hold, then breathe in and return to the first position.

Repetitions: 3 on each side

Full Bend Variation

(pictured, p. 37)

Lace your fingers together behind your back and straighten your arms as much as possible. Breathe in, then breathe out and bend forward, pulling your arms away from your body as far as you can without strain. Tuck your head. Breathe in and return to a standing position.

Repetitions: 3

EXERCISES: 8 MINUTES

Standing Sun Pose *(pictured, p. 44)*

Stand straight, arms at your sides, feet parallel. Breathe out completely. Breathe in and raise your arms to the sides and overhead in a circular motion, press your palms together, and look up. Now start to breathe out, tuck your head, and bend forward from the waist, so your back stays straight as long as possible. Bend forward as far as you can, grasp your ankles or calves with both hands, arms close to your body, then bend your elbows and pull your upper body in toward your legs. Tuck your head. Release, start to breathe in and come up, bringing your arms out to the sides and overhead. Look up, then breathe out and lower your arms to the sides.

Repetitions: 3

Tree Pose (pictured, p. 45)

Stand next to a chair or wall so you can hold on for balance if necessary. Fix your gaze on one spot on the wall in front of you and slowly bring your right foot up on the inside of your left thigh. Consciously relaxing your stomach and your breath, slowly raise both arms over your head, straighten your arms, and press your palms together. Make sure your breath is relaxed. Hold for 10 to 15 seconds, breathing normally. Then release and lower your leg.

Repetitions: 1 on each side

Corpse Pose

Lie on your back with your arms at your sides, close to your body, palms up. Let your feet fall apart slightly. Close your eyes and relax your entire body. Let your breathing relax. Think nothing. Rest for at least a minute.

Knee Squeeze

Improves digestion; limbers and relaxes lower back and hips; improves circulation in pelvic region

Lie on your back with arms over your head on the floor. Breathe out completely. Breathe in and lift your left leg and your head, wrapping your arms around the knee (F). Hold your breath in and squeeze your knee to your chest. Hold for a few seconds, then release, breathe out, and lower the leg and arm back to the starting position. Repeat with the right leg.

Repetitions: 3 on each side

Now do three more repetitions, lifting both legs and your head (G), with the same breath pattern.

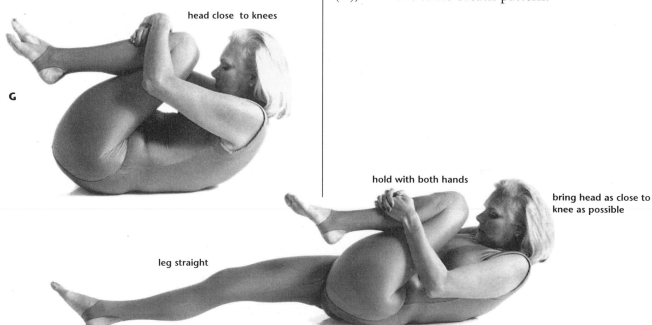

G

head close to knees

hold with both hands

bring head as close to knee as possible

leg straight

F

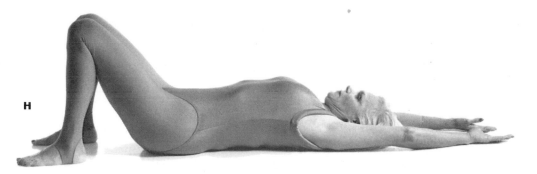

H

Upper Body Stretch with Lock

Limbers shoulders and upper back; prevents incontinence; strengthens lower back and stomach

Lie on your back with arms overhead and knees bent. Separate your feet about 12 inches. Breathe in and stretch your arms and upper torso, then breathe out completely and contract the muscles of your pelvic area (H). Hold for a few seconds, then release.

Repetitions: 3

your elbows on or above your thighs. Breathe in completely, then breathe out as you lean forward slightly and press down on your thighs with your arms (I). Release and repeat twice. Now lace your fingers around your toes, breathe in, and straighten your spine (J). Breathe out as you bend forward, letting your elbows fall *outside* your legs this time (K). Hold for a few seconds, then breathe in and come back up.

Repetitions: 3

Diamond Pose

Sit straight with knees bent and the soles of your feet touching. Grasp your ankles with both hands and rest

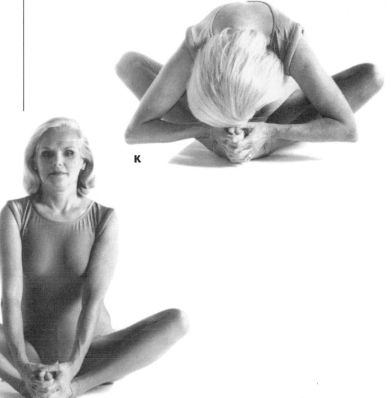

I

J

K

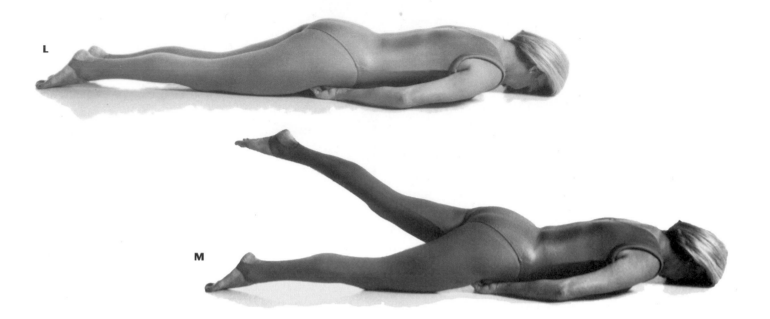

Half Locust

Strengthens spinal column, hips, and legs; improves circulation; improves functioning of digestive system

Lie on your stomach with your forehead on the floor. Make fists and place them just under your hipbones with the thumb end of your fist on the floor (L). Breathe out completely, then breathe in and lift your left leg as high as you can without straining, keeping the knee straight (M). Breathe out, lower the leg, and relax. Repeat with the right leg.

Repetitions: 3 on each side

Easy Bridge *(pictured, p. 49)*

Lie on your back with knees bent and feet several inches apart. Place your hands, palms down, next to your body, or grasp your ankles. Relax your neck and shoulders, breathe in and lift your hips, arching your back. Hold a moment, then breathe out and lower.

Repetitions: 3

MEDITATION: 8 MINUTES

For a review of relaxation and meditation procedures, see Chapter 5. During menopause, daily relaxation and meditation allow you to rest and build focused awareness, which gives you an inner strength and stability that will support you throughout any and every change in your life. Choose a comfortable position and stick with it.

8

TONING AND SHAPING WITH YOGA

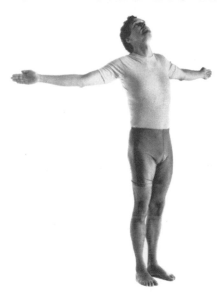

One of the physical benefits of Yoga is a gradual toning and shaping of the body. Though it won't take off inches as fast as more vigorous exercise, Yoga will affect your shape in other ways, such as improving your posture, that you will start to notice within a week or two. Yoga not only tones the body, it tones the emotional personality as well, giving you a steady source of support. Because of the gentle daily discipline and the changes in the breath, you'll begin to like yourself better and feel more creative and energetic. If you are sports-minded, a 20-minute workout can add more depth to your fitness routine by supplementing your physical conditioning with some training in self-awareness. Using Yoga techniques before and after vigorous exercise helps to protect the body from injury because they gently awaken the muscles and change the breath, providing a safe transition into and out of intense activity. This chapter includes two 20-minute workouts that build strength, stamina, and flexibility. Because these workouts are more strenuous than the basic workout, practice the basic workout for at least 2 weeks before you try the workouts in this chapter.

Yoga as Part of a Weight-Loss Program

Yoga can sharpen your concentration, improve your willpower, and help you feel better about yourself as you follow a weight-loss program. You'll feel more attractive while you diet, and you'll find that you can be happy while being self-disciplined. The exercise segment of the 20-minute workout in this chapter is more vigorous than the regular routine, and emphasizes back strengthening, large muscle toning, and shaping of some troublesome areas like the waist, throat, and stomach.

POSTURE

One of the ways Yoga shapes you up is by improving posture. Many of the movements in the exercise portion of your workout stretch and strengthen the postural muscles, lengthening the spine and preventing a humped back. Improved posture will change the way you walk. Another way to improve posture is to practice a seated position. If you can sit comfortably on the floor, supported by cushions, for your seated breathing exercises, practice sitting like that at other times of the day, such as while watching television. You'll strengthen your postural muscles and limber your lower back, hips, and knees at the same time.

CONCENTRATION

Yoga shapes you up by sharpening your concentration. Most people have an average attention span of only about 9 seconds. That's one of the reasons why the camera angles in a film or a television program change so fast. When you divide 9 seconds into the number of hours we are awake each day,

that translates into an immense number of scattered thoughts!

Most of life is like those 9-second sound bites. Not only do we have a lot going on each day, but the constant bombardment of information from the media competes for our attention. We have radios in our cars; Muzak in the stores; stereos, radios, and television (often more than one) at home—is it any wonder that we feel it is unnatural and difficult to concentrate on just one thing for several minutes at a stretch?

This fractured condition prevents us from getting what we want out of life. It causes a piecemeal, disconnected, surface functioning instead of the solid confidence of a person whose concentration is not split. Yoga practice teaches you how to hold your attention on one thing for longer and longer periods. By developing the ability for sustained concentration, you will achieve what you want more quickly. For instance, if you want to lose weight, you need to pay attention to that desire for a great part of every day: you have to consider everything you put into your mouth, you have to stick with an exercise program, you have to be sure that your program is nonviolent to your body, and you have to keep your goal in front of you. Yoga gives you the tools to sustain this intense concentration.

The 20-Minute Workout for Toning and Shaping

BREATHING: 2 MINUTES

Arched Breath (pictured, p. 27)

In a kneeling position, breathe in as you arch forward, breathe out as you round backward.

Repetitions: 3

Complete Breath (full description, pp. 28–29)

In a comfortable seated position, breathe in from the belly up, breathe out from the chest down.

Repetitions: 5-10

Standing 8-Count Breath (full description, p. 30)

Straighten your legs, massaging knees and ankles if necessary. Then stand up and continue breathing evenly to a count of 8 (or begin with 5).

Repetitions: 3

WARMING UP: 2 MINUTES

Follow the regular warm-up routine described on pages 34–38, but substitute the Throat Stretch (pictured and described, page 84) for the Head Roll.

EXERCISE: 8 MINUTES

Because this is a more vigorous routine, you may need to rest more often than normal. Use either the Baby Pose (see page 46) or the Corpse Pose (page 50).

Hip Rock and Rotation (pictured, p. 85)

Stand with feet apart as far as is comfortable, hands on hips with thumbs forward, so fingers support lower back. Gently rotate hips forward and back, side to side, then in circles in both directions. Don't strain or pull.

Repetitions: 3 forward and back, 3 side to side, 3 circles in each direction

Windmill

Limbers and strengthens lower back, hip joints, and upper thighs; improves respiration; reduces waistline

Stand with your feet as far apart as you can comfortably, toes pointed in. Place your hands on your lower back, thumbs over your hips and fingers supporting your lower back. Breathe in completely and turn toward the left. Breathe out as you bend your head and torso toward your left leg (A) and continue moving over to your right leg. Now start to breathe in as you come back to a standing position and face front. Breathe in completely. Repeat twice in the same direction. Your breathing pattern in this exercise follows the movement of your head: if your head moves in a circle, you are breathing out for two-thirds of the circle (from standing, over to the left leg, then to the right leg) and breathing in for the remaining third of the circle (as you stand up).

Repetitions: 3 on each side

A

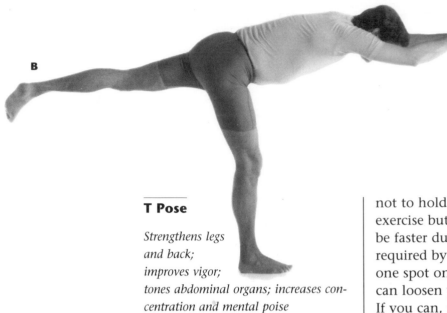

B

T Pose

Strengthens legs and back; improves vigor; tones abdominal organs; increases concentration and mental poise

Start by holding on to a sturdy chair or counter for support until you get more confident. Stand about 3 feet away from the support and lean forward. Balance on your left leg and raise your right leg to the back, parallel to the floor or as high as you can (see top photo, page 116). It's important

not to hold your breath in this exercise but to let it relax; it will be faster due to the extra exertion required by this pose. Staring at one spot on the floor, see if you can loosen your grip on the chair. If you can, raise your arms straight in front of you and place your palms together (B). At first, keep your neck straight and look at a spot on the floor for balance. Later, you can try looking ahead over your thumbs. Hold as long as you can comfortably. Do not strain.

Repetitions: 1 on each side

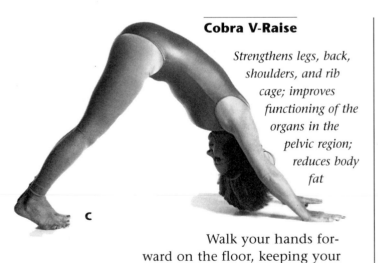

C

Cobra V-Raise

Strengthens legs, back, shoulders, and rib cage; improves functioning of the organs in the pelvic region; reduces body fat

Walk your hands forward on the floor, keeping your heels down as far as possible, until

your hands are about 4 to 5 feet ahead of your feet. Tuck your head and breathe out (C). This is the "V" position. Now, keeping your arms straight, breathe in and slowly lower your body, arching your back and looking up and back (D) (the Cobra position). Push back slowly into the V position, breathing out and tucking your head.

Repetitions: 3

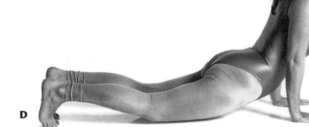

D

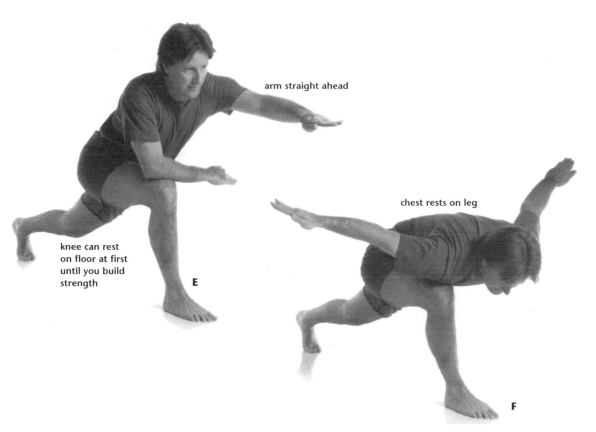

arm straight ahead

knee can rest
on floor at first
until you build
strength

E

chest rests on leg

F

Lunge Sequence

*Strengthens and tones legs and back;
limbers hips and groin muscles*

Throughout this exercise, let your breath take a natural pattern—it will be faster than normal due to the extra exertion required by the exercise. Stand with feet a comfortable distance apart and turn toward the right. Lunge forward on your right foot, resting on the toes of your left (back) foot, and place your hands on either side of your right foot. Rest your right arm on your right knee and extend your left arm straight in front of you (E). Hold for a few seconds. Remember not to hold your breath. Next, extend arms out to your sides, resting your chest on your knee in an "airplane" position (F); hold for a few seconds. Finally, bring both arms down to

the floor on the inside of your right leg, resting your elbows on the floor if you can (G). (If your hips are too stiff for this variation, rest on your hands and just lower your upper body as far as possible.) Hold for a few seconds. Gently straighten up, swivel to the left, and repeat the entire sequence over the left leg.

Repetitions: 1 sequence on each side

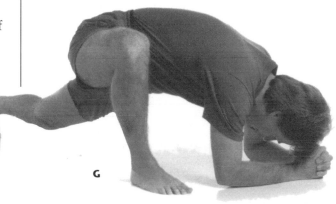

G

Baby Pose *(pictured, p. 46)*

Sit on your feet, bend forward, and rest your head on the floor. Bend your elbows so they rest on the floor. Relax completely, breathing gently, for at least 1 minute.

Seated Sun Pose

Stretches back of legs; limbers and strengthens lower back; massages internal organs

Sit straight with both legs stretched in front, toes flexed back toward your face, arms at your sides. Breathe in as you lift your arms to the sides and overhead. Look up and stretch, elongating your spine (H). Then breathe out and bend forward over your legs, tucking your head. Grasp your ankles with both hands (or, if you can reach your toes *comfortably*, grasp the toes as shown on page 48).

arms straight up

back straight

toes flexed

H

Bend your arms and pull gently (I). Hold for a few seconds. Then release, breathe in, and bring your arms in another circle to the sides and overhead. Look up. Breathe out and lower your arms to your sides.

Repetitions: 3

I

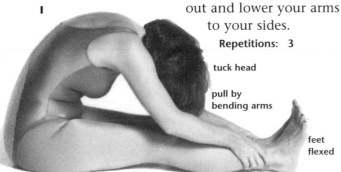

tuck head

pull by bending arms

feet flexed

knees straight

Front Crow *(pictured, p. 66)*

Squat on your toes and place your hands on the floor between your knees, about a foot apart. Bend your elbows and place the inside joints of your knees on your elbows. Holding that position, carefully lean forward, resting your bent legs on the back of your elbows, until your feet come off the floor. Don't hold your breath; let your body decide how to breathe. Hold the position for at least 5 seconds if you can.

Repetitions: 1

Big Sit-up

Strengthens abdominal and thigh muscles; improves balance and concentration

Lie on your back with arms overhead. Breathe out. Breathe in, then lift both arms, both legs, and upper body so you are balancing on your buttocks. Reach for your toes, keeping your legs straight, and try to touch your toes (J). Relax and breathe out, returning to the starting position.

Repetitions: 3

J

Boat Pose

Strengthens back muscles; improves digestion and functioning of all internal organs

Lie on your stomach, forehead to the floor and arms stretched out in

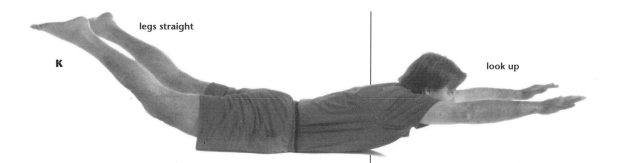

legs straight

K

look up

front. Breathe out, then breathe in and lift your arms, legs, and head (K). Look up. Hold for a second, then breathe out and lower back to the starting position.

Repetitions: 3

RELAXATION AND MEDITATION: 8 MINUTES

For a review of the relaxation and meditation procedures, see Chapter 5.

Yoga and Sports

Here is a 20-minute workout for those of you who follow a regular sports program. Yoga can add a new depth to any fitness routine, because the emphasis in Yoga is not solely on physical conditioning. When most people exercise, they are thinking about something else. When you make a 20-minute Yoga workout part of your routine, you'll find not only physical conditioning but also concentration, strength, stamina, and enjoyment. Try a fantasy technique to enhance your sports performance and experience. If you are a runner, for instance, picture in your mind how your ideal runner looks and feels. Spend several minutes concentrating on that picture. Then, when you run, think about what you are doing. Hear your heart beat. Enjoy the feelings in your muscles. Be conscious of your breathing. Feel the wind on your face and the pavement under your feet. Become that runner you fantasize about.

Don't wait for the "runner's high"; create your own by making your exercise part of you, not just an appendage to your life. You'll find a great deal more enjoyment in any exercise program when you approach it wholeheartedly and bring it into your mind as well as your body.

Because so many people run or lift weights, the exercise portion of the following 20-minute workout concentrates on exercises that stretch and relax the body.

BREATHING: 2 MINUTES

Arched Breath *(pictured, p. 27)*

In a kneeling position, breathe in as you arch forward, breathe out as you round backward.

Repetitions: 3

Complete Breath (full description, pp. 28–29)

In a comfortable seated position, breathe in from the belly up, breathe out from the chest down.

Repetitions: 5-10

Standing 8-Count Breath (full description, p. 30)

Straighten your legs, massaging knees and ankles if necessary. Then stand up and continue breathing evenly to a count of 8 (or begin with 5).

Repetitions: 3

WARMING UP: 2 MINUTES

Follow the routine outlined in Chapter 3.

EXERCISE: 8 MINUTES

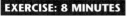

Full Bend

Improves respiration and posture; limbers legs and lower back muscles

Stand with feet parallel, arms at your sides. Breathe in completely as you raise your arms out to the sides and then back (L). Breathe out and bend forward from the waist as far as you can, keeping your knees straight. At the bottom, let your hands, arms, and head relax completely and just hang for a few seconds. Breathe in and stand up, bringing your arms back to the outstretched position.

L

Immediately breathe out and bend forward again, so the exercise is one continuous up-and-down motion.

Repetitions: 5-10

Hip Rock and Rotation (pictured, p. 85)

Stand with feet as far apart as is comfortable, hands on hips with thumbs forward, so fingers support lower back. Gently rotate hips forward and back, then side to side, then in circles in each direction. Don't strain or pull.

Repetitions: 3 forward and back, 3 side to side, 3 circles in each direction

Windmill (pictured, p. 91)

Stand with your feet as far apart as you can comfortably, toes pointed in. Place your hands on your lower back, thumbs over your hips and fingers supporting your lower back. Start by breathing in completely and turning toward the left. Breathe out as you bend toward your left leg and as you continue moving over to your right leg. Now start to breathe in as you come back to a standing position and face front. Breathe in completely. Your breathing pattern in this exercise follows the movement of your head: if your head moves in a circle, you are breathing out for two-thirds of the circle (from standing, over to the left leg, then to the right leg) and breathing in for the remaining third of the circle (as you stand up).

Repetitions: 3 in each direction

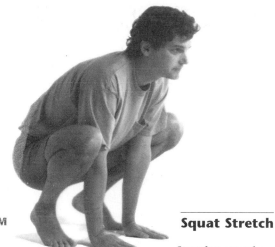

M

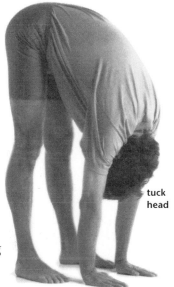

straighten
knees as much
as possible

tuck
head

N

Squat Stretch

Stretches muscles and nerves in the back of the legs; limbers lower back

Squat with feet slightly apart and hands on the floor between and slightly in front of your feet (the closer to your feet, the greater the stretch). Breathe in, looking for-ward (M), then breathe out and straighten your legs as much as possible without straining, tucking your head (N). Breathe in and return to your starting position.

Repetitions: 3

T Pose Knee Bend

Strengthens back and knee joints

Holding on to a sturdy chair or counter for support, lower your torso and raise your left leg in back so it's parallel to the floor or as high as you can. Loosen your grip on the chair and slowly bring your hands back to clasp the fingers loosely over your back (O). Stare at one spot on the floor for balance, and don't hold your breath. Carefully bend your right leg without allowing your torso or your left leg to fall from their parallel position (P). Then slowly straighten.

Repetitions: 3-5

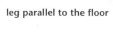

leg parallel to the floor

knee straight

O

keep leg and torso
parallel to the floor

P

Thigh Stretch

Stretches all muscles of the legs and hips; improves respiration

Stand with feet a comfortable distance apart and swivel to face right. Bend forward and place your hands on either side of your right foot. Bend your right leg, lower your hips, breathe in, arch your back, and look up (Q).

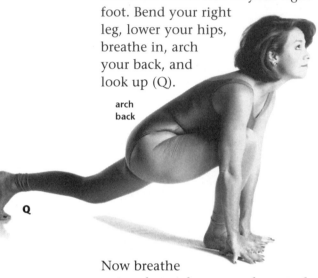

arch back

Q

Now breathe out and straighten your legs, tucking your head in toward your right leg (R). Keep the toes of your right foot pointed. Repeat twice over the right leg, then stand up and swivel in the opposite direction.

Repetitions: 3 on each side

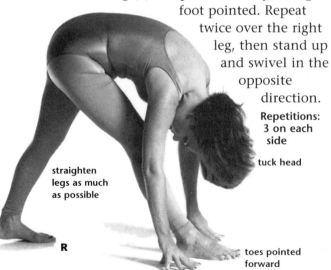

straighten legs as much as possible

R

tuck head

toes pointed forward

Baby Pose *(pictured, p. 46)*

Fold over in a kneeling position so your head rests on the floor and your arms rest at your sides. Let your elbows fall outward. Breathe gently. Rest for at least a minute.

Limber Hips

Limbers hip and knee joints

Seated with both legs stretched in front of you, carefully lift your right foot with both hands and place the ankle on your left thigh. Lean back on your left hand and press down gently on the right knee with your right hand (S). Press and release several times. Use your hands to carefully lower the leg and switch sides.

Repetitions: 5-6 on each side

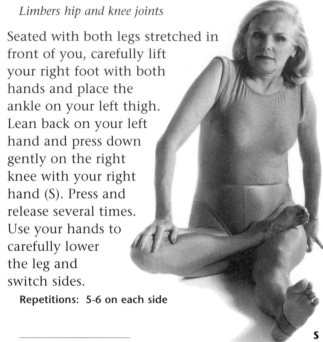

S

Seated Sun Pose

(pictured, p. 94)

Sit straight with both legs stretched in front, toes pulled back toward your face, arms at your sides. Breathe in as you lift your arms to the sides and overhead. Look up and stretch, elongating your spine. Then breathe out and bend forward over your legs, tucking your head. Grasp your ankles with both hands (or, if you can reach your toes *comfortably*, grasp the toes as shown on page 48). Bend your arms and pull gently. Hold for a few seconds. Then release, breathe in, and bring your arms in a circle to the sides and overhead. Look up. Breathe out and lower your arms to your sides.

Repetitions: 3

Tortoise Stretch *(pictured, p. 47)*

Sit with legs separated as far as possible. Pull your feet back toward your face, lean back on your hands, lift your hips slightly, and push your pelvis forward. Then sit straight, rest your hands on your legs, and point your toes. Hold for a few seconds.

Repetitions: 2

Then, with feet flexed again, breathe in and raise your arms in a circle over your head. Look up. Now breathe out and bend toward your left leg. Grasp the ankle or calf with both hands and bend your elbows slightly, pulling your upper body *gently* toward your legs. Keep your knees straight. Your breath should be completely out. Hold for a few seconds, then breathe in, raise your arms in a circular motion overhead, look up, then breathe out and lower your arms in another circle to your sides.

Repetitions: 3 on each side

Finally, reach forward and grasp the calves, ankles, or toes with both hands and hold, breathing gently, for several seconds.

Repetitions: 1

Shoulder Stand *(pictured, p. 68)*

If you have a disk problem in your neck, do not do this exercise. Substitute the Easy Bridge (pictured page 49) instead. Hold this pose as long as you can comfortably. Start by sitting with knees drawn up to chest and arms wrapped around knees. Gently roll back and forth a few times to make sure that the spine is in place with no pinched nerves or strained muscles. Then roll back, keeping knees to forehead, and immediately support your back with your hands. Hold this position until you feel steady, then slowly straighten your legs. If your legs appear to be more at a 45° angle, move your hands down your back toward the floor and tuck your chin into your chest; your legs should straighten a bit more. Fix your gaze on the space between your big toes. Relax your breath. Hold as long as you can comfortably. Come out of the pose by bending your knees and bringing them to your forehead. Slowly roll forward, rounding your back, until you come all the way up to a seated position. Bend forward for a few seconds to be sure the blood doesn't drain from your head too fast.

Repetitions: 1

Fish Pose

Limbers and strengthens back and neck; improves eyesight; improves posture

Lie on your back with arms at your sides. Bend your elbows slightly and arch your back so you are resting on the top of your head (T). Stare at one spot and do not blink. You can use your arms to help with the support, but try to use primarily your back muscles. Look up into your forehead and hold the position for several seconds, breathing normally.

Repetitions: 1

stare at one spot—don't blink

T

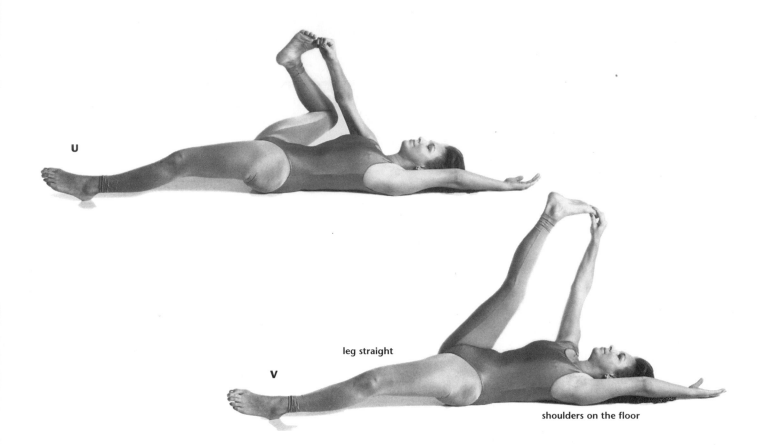

U

leg straight

V

shoulders on the floor

Extra Leg Stretch

Strengthens legs and back; limbers legs and hips

Lie on your back with arms overhead. Grasp your right big toe with your right hand (U) and straighten your leg as much as possible (V). Hold a few seconds. Repeat with left leg.

Repetitions: 1 on each side

RELAXATION AND MEDITATION: 8 MINUTES

For a review of the relaxation and meditation procedures, see Chapter 5.

9

THE 20-MINUTE WORKOUT WHEN YOU'RE NOT AT HOME

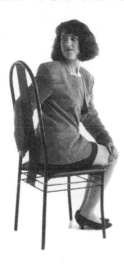

Sometimes you can't be at home for your regular 20-minute workout. The demands of travel and business often change your schedule and take you away from the familiar surroundings where you've created a daily discipline for your Yoga practice. If you find yourself spending a lot of time away from the same room, or even the same city, the workout variations and suggestions in this chapter will help you create the atmosphere needed for your regular daily 20-minute practice of Yoga wherever you may be.

Yoga as Part of the Workday

Many people have a limited—and often negative—idea about work. Part of the definition of being an American, it seems, is someone who is always working. Traditionally, in this country, we take very little time on a regular basis to refresh ourselves in stillness. In Yoga, that regular time of stillness is seen as a way to work on yourself; you take time in every day to refresh your body and mind with creative thought and experience. Yoga is a type of work that helps you work; as such, it is needed during work time. Try expanding your definition of work. Give yourself this 20-minute gift every day, and you will be boosting your capabilities by injecting balance and new energy into your life.

If you're something of a workaholic, and you find yourself spending more time at work than at home, put your 20-minute workout into your workday. If you don't have a private office or a room where you can shut the door, you'll have to improvise: do a few exercises and breathing tech-

TRANSITION AND REENTRY

When you have an active lifestyle and a full schedule, it's important to give some conscious attention to *transition* and *reentry* between activities. Otherwise, you will always feel scattered and not altogether there—as though your mind cannot catch up with your body. This transition should be restful and a real change from what you were doing previously. If you're going from one job to another, or when you've just come home from work, take a few minutes to do something that is not work and that does not involve interacting with others: sit down and read a magazine; have a cold drink; take a short nap; do some Yoga. If you have the time and the facilities, water is the best way to change your mood and thought: a quick shower, a dip in the pool—even washing your hands and sprinkling some water on your head. You can use Yoga as part of that reentry. If you don't have time to do a full 20-minute workout, pick a few techniques to remind yourself of how you feel when you practice. When you do have time for a full 20-minute workout, you'll find that it refreshes and energizes you so you can go full steam ahead with whatever you have to do.

niques at your desk, and then head for the bathroom, lock the door, and spend a few minutes on meditation. Nobody will complain about the time, and you'll have a few minutes of privacy to relax and quiet your mind. Some of my students have even persuaded their employers to provide a spare room for a quick "meditation" break during the day.

What Yoga provides in the 20-minute routine at work is a way to change your thinking. Sometimes, in the middle of the day, you suddenly "surface," feeling drained, fatigued, wiped out. Minutes or hours have gone by in deep concentration, and you've forgotten everything except what you're working on. At those times, your breath becomes shallower, and less and less oxygen gets to your brain. Suddenly you feel almost suffocated. That's the time to take a break: do some deep diaphragmatic breathing and move around a little to increase circulation so your brain gets some nutrients. At the same time, change your thinking, rattle your brain waves, stimulate the areas of intuition and creativity that may have been pushed aside by all that wonderful logical business-world thinking, and give yourself the gift of some new ideas.

The 20-Minute Workout at Work

Get up from your desk, go into the bathroom, and wash your hands. Sprinkle a few drops of water over your head, pretending you are standing in a cool, fresh rain, and declare yourself changed. Water has the ability to change your mental environment. Make sure no one is going to disturb you for your 20 minutes. Ask for your calls to be held, or turn off your phone and turn on your voice mail.

Then go back to your desk and start with 2 minutes of breathing. The Arched Breath (page 27) will get you to use your diaphragm more, limber and release tension in your lower back, and get your mind off business and onto what's happening right now. Then do a few repetitions of the Complete Breath (page 28). Concentrate on the sound of the breath, until it becomes the only thing in your mind; the only thing in existence for you at this moment. This will immediately start refreshing your mind because the tensions and concerns of the day will fade to

the background, and the frantic whirling of thoughts will cease.

Now stand up and do a few more Complete Breaths, feeling the fresh oxygen and energy reaching down to your toes and up into your head. Count to 8 when you breathe in; count to 8 when you breathe out. When you breathe out, think of the tension and fatigue draining out with the breath. Use your imagination to see and feel stress leaving you. Then replace it with energy and strength.

This fantasy technique is very important in removing stress from the body. The use of fantasy brings the mind back to itself; it helps you stop thinking of other people and other things. Continue using

---

HOW MEDITATION UNLOCKS CREATIVITY AND INTUITION

Meditation can release certain facets of your mind that usually remain in the background. These wonderful qualities are like shy cousins; they stay away from the constant clamor and volley of thought, emotional reaction, and sensory perception. They reside in every person's mind, but they come out only when they are welcomed with quietness, awareness, and observation. They are creativity and intuition.

Sometimes you will notice that in the middle of a quiet, attentive meditation, the answer to a problem at work or home will suddenly appear. You might be reminded of times when you've gone to bed worrying about something and awakened with the clear answer. By temporarily "turning off" your limited, conscious mind, you allow your subconscious to present the solution to you. The same happens in meditation. You stop thinking momentarily, and then the truth can emerge.

Intuition appears not dramatically, like a voice out of the sky, but as a feeling that you gradually become aware of. You can see how important it is to have some training in quietness for this to be able to happen. There are ways to practice listening for intuition—little games you can play all day: for instance, when you're driving to work, see if you can notice a feeling about which lane of traffic will move fastest. Or when the telephone rings, do you have a feeling of who it is? These feelings can serve you if you cultivate them and become more aware of their presence.

fantasy as you do the following exercises. The exercise segment in this 20-minute workout includes movements that are designed to work out kinks in the upper back and neck, to improve circulation to the head, to relieve lower back tension, and to release tense stomach muscles. The poor posture that arises during the afternoon hours is usually due to upper back muscles that are hot and fatigued. The poses that squeeze the shoulder blades together or bend the body backward are especially useful for removing fatigue.

The first four exercises can be done either standing or seated. If you work at a keyboard, you will benefit from doing these exercises several times a day.

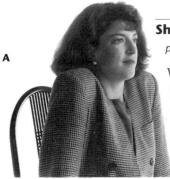

A

Shoulder Roll *(full description, p. 34)*

With your arms loose at your sides, lift your shoulders toward your ears (A) and roll them forward several times, then back several times.

Repetitions: 3-4 in each direction

Arm Roll *(pictured, p. 35)*

Stretch arms out to the sides with palms facing outward and elbows straight. Rotate them in large circles, then smaller circles.

Repetitions: 3-4 large circles in each direction, 4-5 small circles in each direction

Head Rock

Relax your shoulders and bend your head forward. Rotate your head slowly to one side (ear over the shoulder, not your chin), then down in front again and over to the other side. Continue rolling your head back and forth in a half circle for several repetitions.

Repetitions: 5-6

B

Elbow Touch *(full description, p. 79)*

Bring your fingers to your shoulders, breathe out, and touch your elbows together in front. Breathe in and move your elbows toward the back as far as you can (B).

Repetitions: 5-10

Full Bend Variation *(pictured, p. 37)*

Slip your shoes off if you are wearing heels. Stand with feet parallel and clasp your hands behind you. Straighten your arms as much as possible. Breathe in completely, then breathe out and bend forward, pulling your arms away from your body and keeping your knees straight. Tuck your chin. Breathe in and come back to a standing position.

Repetitions: 3

Full Bend Hold *(pictured, p. 37)*

Bend forward from the waist and let your head and arms hang loosely down. Keep knees straight. Breathe normally and hold for several seconds.

Repetitions: 1

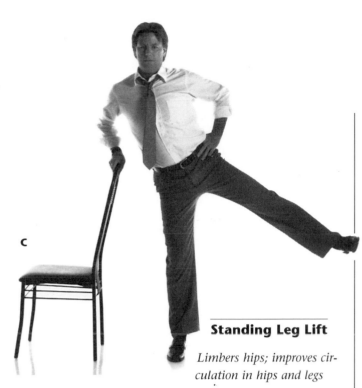

C

Standing Leg Lift

Limbers hips; improves circulation in hips and legs

If you are wearing heels, slip off your shoes for this exercise. Hold on to a chair with your right hand for support and stare at one spot for balance. Put your left hand on your left hip and lift your left leg forward while breathing in. Breathe out and lower. Repeat to the side (C) and to the back.

Repetitions: 3 in each direction with each leg

Standing Reach *(pictured, p. 84, top left)*

Breathe out completely with arms at your sides. Breathe in and raise your arms out to the sides and overhead in a circular motion. Stretch up. Breathe out and lower arms.

Repetitions: 3

Standing Twist

Improves balance, concentration, and poise; strengthens legs and feet; improves respiration

Breathe out completely with arms at your sides. Breathe in and raise your arms in a circular motion overhead. Press your palms together. Hold your breath in and slowly twist your torso to the left (D). Return to the front, breathe out, and lower your arms to your sides. Repeat to the other side.

Repetitions: 3 on each side

Baby Pose

Sit with your hips against the back of your chair. Bend forward and rest your folded arms on your knees. Let your head relax. If it is comfortable, let your arms fall below your knees so your upper body is lying across your legs (E). Completely relax and hold for 30 seconds to 1 minute. This is another wonderful exercise for bringing fresh blood and the nutrients it carries to the brain.

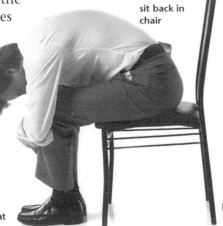

sit back in chair

let head and neck relax

feet flat

D

E

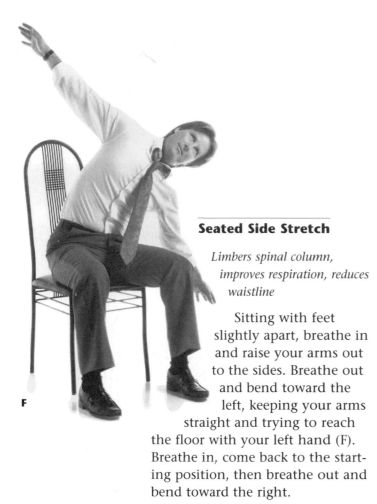

F

Seated Leg Lifts

Strengthens legs, hips, and lower back; improves circulation to legs and feet

Hold on to the seat of your chair for leverage. Breathe out, then breathe in as you lift your right leg straight, foot flexed (G). Breathe out and lower your leg.

Repetitions: 3 for each leg

Seated Side Stretch

Limbers spinal column, improves respiration, reduces waistline

Sitting with feet slightly apart, breathe in and raise your arms out to the sides. Breathe out and bend toward the left, keeping your arms straight and trying to reach the floor with your left hand (F). Breathe in, come back to the starting position, then breathe out and bend toward the right.

Repetitions: 3 on each side

Ankle Rotations and Point-Flexes

Improves circulation to feet

Hold on to the seat of your chair, stretch your legs out in front of you, and rotate your ankles several times in each direction. Then point and flex the feet several times.

Repetitions: 5-6 circles in each direction, 5-6 point-flexes

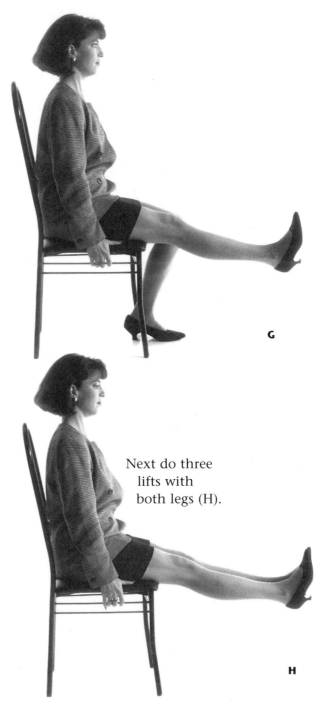

G

Next do three lifts with both legs (H).

H

look to right
and
slightly up

sit straight

pull with
left hand

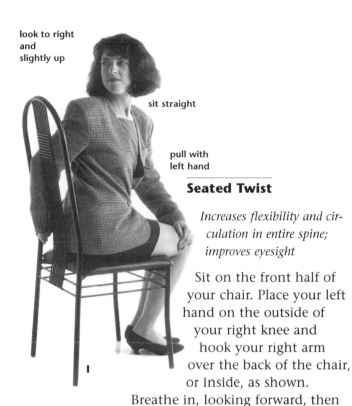

Seated Twist

Increases flexibility and circulation in entire spine; improves eyesight

Sit on the front half of your chair. Place your left hand on the outside of your right knee and hook your right arm over the back of the chair, or inside, as shown. Breathe in, looking forward, then breathe out as you twist to the right. Turn your head and eyes as far right as they will go and stare at a spot just above eye level (I). Pull slightly on your right knee with your left hand for more leverage. Relax your breath and hold the position, breathing normally, for several seconds. Release and repeat on the opposite side.

Repetitions: 1 on each side

bring head to
knee as far as
possible

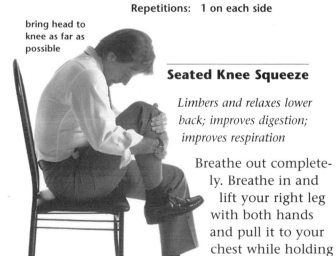

Seated Knee Squeeze

Limbers and relaxes lower back; improves digestion; improves respiration

Breathe out completely. Breathe in and lift your right leg with both hands and pull it to your chest while holding your breath in. Tuck your head

toward your knee and let your raised foot relax (J). Hold for a few seconds, then release and switch sides.

Repetitions: 3 on each side

Sun Pose in Chair

Improves circulation to head; massages internal organs; limbers spine and hip joints

Separate your legs and sit with your hips against the back of the chair. Breathe out completely. Breathe in and raise your arms in a circle to the sides and overhead. Look up and stretch (K). Breathe out, tuck your head, and bend forward between your legs. If you can reach the floor, place your palms flat (L). Breathe in and raise your arms up over your head again, then breathe out and lower your arms to the sides.

Repetitions: 3

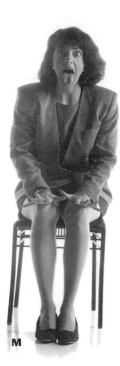

Lion

Relaxes facial muscles; relieves anxiety and depression; changes mood

Sit comfortably with hands on your knees. Take a deep breath in, then breathe out quickly with a growling sound as you open your eyes and mouth wide, stick out your tongue, and tense your fingers (M).

Repetitions: 3 (or as needed)

Finish with relaxation and meditation, seated, with a cushion at your lower back if your chair doesn't properly support your lower back. It is often difficult to go from much mental activity to nothing—even when you're at home, relaxed, and comfortable. At work it may be even harder. Try not to judge how you're doing. Remember, you don't really know what meditation is supposed to feel like; you only know that your immediate goal is to momentarily stop talking to yourself. Even if the mental conversation stops for only a few seconds, notice how it feels, and then try for it again. During your meditation period, try to put all thoughts of work out of your mind.

If your office is a bit noisy, use fantasy to help turn inward. Imagine the sound blending into one low hum in the background and gradually getting fainter. Imagine yourself on the other side of a glass wall from the sound, so you physically disconnect from it. Mentally turn your attention away from the work sounds into yourself, toward your inner being, your source of strength, power, and creativity.

When your meditation period is over, gently stretch, slowly start to move around, and give yourself a minute or so to think about how you feel. How is this feeling different from the way you ordinarily feel when you're at work? Notice the change. If you can remember the different feeling, you'll be able to re-create it whenever you want it, throughout the day. Each time you remember how you feel in meditation, even if you are going full steam ahead in your work, you'll have a few seconds of a different thought, a different feeling, and that makes whatever else you do during the day fresh and creative.

Travel

If you're on the move a great deal, and you truly want to develop the habit of daily practice, you'll probably need to vary your routine now and then to adapt to your changing schedule and environment.

Even if you don't enjoy travel, it's difficult to keep to a steady routine. The stress of airports,

tight schedules, and unfamiliar people and places demands extra attention; on top of that, you may have extra responsibilities, particularly if you're a business traveler. When traveling, you always have to be ready for the unexpected. These extra stresses have a tendency to draw you away from your daily discipline, and it will be necessary to learn how to re-create the atmosphere for your practice wherever you are.

Don't forget your 20-minute workout at these times—this is when you need it most! Put it into your schedule: write it—in ink—on your daily calendar. If you're used to doing your 20-minute workout in the morning, try to maintain that schedule even when you're away from home. It will work best if you choose a time that will be free every day. Many people find that the late afternoon is a very good time to practice. Energy is often low then, and a 20-minute workout will give you some extra energy for the rest of the day and evening. Try it instead of caffeine for a pick-me-up that doesn't let you down later.

If you're on a pleasure trip with family or friends, and don't have your own room, be creative. Be assertive. Ask for 20 minutes all to yourself. Or delay going to a meal with everyone else for a few minutes, and do part of your routine then. If you have to, you can split up your 20-minute workout—do a few exercises before eating, do your breathing while you're lying on the beach, and take 10 minutes in the bathroom for your meditation.

HOW TO CREATE A HOME AWAY FROM HOME FOR YOGA

Take your blanket or mat with you. When you're in strange surroundings, you need something of your own to help you feel safe and protected. If you like to pack light, designate a thin shawl or half sheet as your "traveling mat." Some students buy 2 or 3 yards of lightweight material that folds into next to nothing and designate that as their traveling Yoga mat. It's important to use something that is your own for exercising, even if the room is carpeted. Just consider how many people have used the room, and you'll realize how necessary it is to put something of your own between you and the floor. Pack your exercise clothes or buy a lightweight pair of pajamas or shorts and a T-shirt and designate that as your traveling exercise outfit. Your Yoga clothes and mat should not be used for anything else. Pack a pair of earplugs (see Chapter 2, pages 25–26). Make sure your room has a "Do Not Disturb" sign, and use it. Put a "Do Not Disturb" order on your phone as well.

Since you have only 20 minutes, make the most of them. Plan ahead so you can quickly reduce the stress of travel and settle into your normal routine.

As soon as you get to your hotel room, head straight for the shower. Unless you have an urgent meeting and can't wait, use the warm water to change your thinking and help you relax. Standing in the shower with hot water on your neck, breathe deeply a few times. You can also do a few simple warm-ups, such as Shoulder Rolls. This is your reentry time; don't think about work or anything else except how you feel right now.

After your shower, put on your exercise clothes, spread out your blanket or mat, and begin. You can use your regular 20-minute workout, or try the variation described on the following pages. The exercises in this routine are designed to release tension in your upper and lower back, work out the kinks of travel, get the circulation going in your entire body, and increase your concentration.

BREATHING: 2 MINUTES

Follow your regular breathing segment (see Chapter 2).

WARMING UP: 2 MINUTES

Follow your regular warm-up sequence (see Chapter 3).

ASANS: 8 MINUTES

Standing Sun Pose (pictured, p. 44)

Stand with feet parallel. Breathe in and raise your arms in a circle overhead. Stretch and look up. Breathe out and bend forward, tucking your head and bending from the waist. Grasp your ankles or calves, bend your elbows, and pull gently. Keep your knees straight. Hold for a few seconds, then release, breathe in, and come back up, bringing your arms in another circle overhead. Breathe out and lower your arms.

Repetitions: 3

Tree Pose (pictured, p. 45)

Stand on your right leg and lift your left foot to rest on the inside of your right thigh as high up as you can. Consciously relax your stomach and your breath. When you feel balanced, slowly raise your arms over your head, palms together. Keep your arms straight. Stare at one spot for balance. Hold for several seconds, then gently lower your left leg and repeat with the right.

Repetitions: 1 on each side

Cat Breath (pictured, p. 74)

On hands and knees, breathe in, arch your back and look up, then breathe out and round your back, pulling in your stomach and tucking your head.

Repetitions: 3

Camel Pose

Limbers entire spine; improves circulation and respiration; stretches and strengthens thighs and knees; improves functioning of thyroid

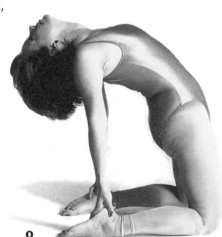

Kneel with legs slightly separated. The first two movements in this exercise help to prepare the spine for an intense stretch. Carefully bend back and grasp your left heel with your left hand. Push your hips forward slightly (N). Repeat on the right side. Now bend backward and grasp both heels. Push your hips forward as far as possible and let your head relax back (O). Hold for several seconds, breathing normally. Release and rest briefly in the Baby Pose.

Repetitions: 1

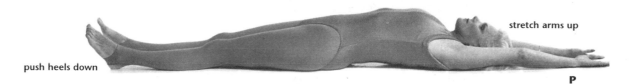

push heels down

stretch arms up

P

Baby Pose *(pictured, p. 46)*

Kneel and bend your head forward to the floor. Let your arms relax to your sides with the elbows on the floor. Relax your breath. Hold for about one minute.

Knee Squeeze *(pictured, p. 86)*

Lying on your back with arms overhead, breathe in and lift one knee toward your chest. Lift your head toward the knee. Hold your breath and pull the knee to your chest with both hands. Release, breathe out, and lower the leg and arms.

Repetitions: 3 on each side, 3 with both legs

Alternate Toe Touch *(pictured, p. 48)*

Lying on your back with arms overhead, breathe in and lift your left arm and leg, foot flexed, and try to touch your toes without lifting your shoulder. Breathe out and lower.

Repetitions: 3 on each side, alternating

Easy Bridge *(pictured, p. 49)*

Lying on your back, bend your knees and separate your feet several inches. Breathe in and raise your hips, arching your back. Keep shoulders and neck relaxed. Breathe out and lower.

Repetitions: 3

Floor Stretch

Limbers and releases tight muscles in entire spine and backs of legs

Lie on the floor with arms overhead (P). Breathe normally. Stretch your left arm upward and left leg downward, keeping feet flexed and pushing your heels away from you. Repeat on the right. Then stretch both arms and legs.

Repetitions: 1 on each side, 1 both together

Knee Swing *(pictured, p. 77)*

Lie on your back with knees bent, feet about 2 feet apart, and arms stretched out to the sides, palms down. Bend both knees to the left, keeping your hips on the floor, then bend them to the right, alternating slowly. Let your breath relax into a natural pattern of breathing out each time your knees go to one side, and breathing in as your knees come back up straight.

Repetitions: 10-20

Cobra Pose *(pictured, p. 46)*

Lie on your stomach with forehead on the floor and hands under your shoulders, palms down, elbows up. Breathe out completely. Breathe in and slowly curl up, starting with your head and eyes, then your chest, then your stomach. Use your back muscles; don't straighten your arms. Breathe out and curl down, starting with the stomach; keep your head and eyes back until the very last.

Repetitions: 3

Corpse Pose

Lie on your back and relax every muscle.

RELAXATION AND MEDITATION: 8 MINUTES

Even if you are used to sitting up for meditation, you might want to meditate lying down for a more restful session while you are traveling.

The Airplane Workout

Here is a challenge. Do you have enough self-confidence to risk the stares of fellow passengers as you do some small exercises in your coach seat? You can very creatively get in a few exercises, some breathing, and some meditation while you're traveling. Carry my meditation tape in your briefcase (see Appendix); time flies by as you meditate, and you will arrive at your destination refreshed instead of fatigued, relaxed instead of stiff, and ready for whatever you have to face at the end of your journey.

Breathing is your best tool for dealing with the stress of travel. You've probably experienced the drowsiness and mental dullness from breathing recirculated, stale air. Rhythmic breathing will help you get more oxygen to your brain as well as calm your thoughts.

Start with breathing. Close your eyes and pretend to be sleeping. Sit as straight as you can (sometimes a pillow in the small of your back helps) and breathe for several minutes, concentrating on the sound of your breath.

Do a few exercises. Without attracting too much attention, you can easily do the following exercises:

Seated Knee Squeeze (page 107)

Ankle Rotations and Point-Flexes (page 106)

Shoulder Roll (page 104)

Head Roll (page 35)

A Seated Twist if you have enough room (page 107)

Then settle back for a good long **relaxation and meditation** session (time it so you're not likely to be disturbed by the drinks cart). If you have my cassette tape on meditation, put it in your portable tape player, close your eyes, and relax. If you aren't using the tape, keep your earphones on anyway— it will help reduce the noises around you and others will be less likely to disturb you.

10

THE 20-MINUTE WORKOUT WHEN YOU'RE NOT FEELING YOUR BEST

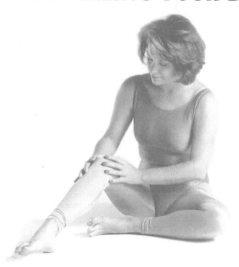

No body is perfect. Most of us occasionally have a joint that aches, or a back problem that nags, or days when we feel slightly under the weather. Sometimes exercise is just what you need. If you are over 30, you need to be sure to exercise as much as you can. Inactivity is responsible for more aches and pains and lethargic feelings than actual diseases are. If you've been injured, you need to start moving again as soon as the pain is gone. Every day of total bed rest results in a percentage loss of muscle tone. Even when you're in the hospital, you'll be urged to get up and start moving right after surgery, even if it's just a walk to the bathroom. No one recommends full bed rest for days and days anymore. It's not healthy.

If you have a physical problem that prevents you from doing the regular 20-minute workout, or on days when you don't feel up to par, alter the exercise segment and increase your meditation time. This chapter presents a few suggestions on how to vary your routine if you aren't feeling your best.

Daily practice is important, so even if you have to modify your routine a great deal, try to do something every day. The continuity of regular practice will tap into your inner strength and help you heal more quickly.

You can use a fantasy technique to enhance the effects of your practice. A great part of the effect of Yoga—even the exercises—happens in your mind. If you're too ill to get out of bed, you can still practice Yoga by fantasizing yourself doing three exercises; visualize yourself doing them with the correct breathing and movements, at the correct speed. Then do some Complete Breaths lying on your back, and extend your meditation time.

Remember: Always check with your doctor or physical therapist before starting any exercise routine, especially if you have a chronic condition.

Back and Neck Problems

Bad backs are very common—about 20% of all adults have some kind of chronic or recurrent problem with the muscles of the back or disks of the spinal column. The most common areas affected are the back of the neck and the lower back, and the most common reason for back problems is a combination of too little exercise, weak muscles, poor posture, and inappropriate office furniture. Some problems are caused by an abnormality in the spinal column that results in disks being herniated or degenerating. Many physicians feel that the gentle stretching and strengthening aspects of Yoga exercises can be good for those who can't do more vigorous exercise because of a bad back. And all physicians will agree that some daily exercise is essential. Exercise prevents weak muscles caused by lack of muscle tone. Weak muscles pull the back out of shape faster. The postural muscles on either side of the spine are especially important to keep in tone.

The following workout is designed to gently strengthen muscles in the back and provide a maintenance program of limberness and strength that will prevent a back problem from worsening and will gradually relieve it. To supplement this program, you should follow the recommended guidelines about the proper way to sit, stand, and lift things (available from any physical therapist, chiropractic physician, or orthopedic physician). Examine the chair you use at work, and make sure that it is of the proper height, with proper back support.

BREATHING: 2 MINUTES

Arched Breath (pictured, p. 27)

In a kneeling position, or sitting on the edge of a chair, place your hands on your knees and breathe out completely. Breathe in, arch your back, and look up. Breathe out, round your back, and tuck your head.

Repetitions: 3

Complete Breath (full description, pp. 28–29)

In a comfortable seated position on the floor or in a chair, breathe in and out evenly and smoothly, concentrating on the sound of the breath.

Repetitions: 5-10

Standing 8-Count Breath (full description, p. 30)

Straighten your legs and carefully stand up. Continue the Complete Breath to a count of 8.

Repetitions: 3

Shoulder Roll (pictured, p. 34)

Keeping your arms loose at your sides, rotate your shoulders forward and back several times. Breathe normally.

Repetitions: 3-4 in each direction

Arm Roll (pictured, p. 35)

Hold your arms straight out with palms facing outward. Rotate your arms in large, slow circles first forward, then backward. Breathe normally.

Repetitions: 3-4 in each direction

Head Tilts

Bend your head forward slowly, then tilt it back carefully. Then tilt to one side, ear over the shoulder, and tilt to the opposite side. Turn and look over your left shoulder, then your right. Always move very carefully. Breathe normally.

Repetitions: 5-6 in each direction

Elbow Touch (pictured, p. 104)

With fingers on your shoulders, breathe out and touch your elbows together in front. Breathe in and stretch your elbows toward the back as far as possible.

Repetitions: 3

Elbow Twist (pictured, p. 36)

Hold your arms in front of you, elbows bent and one hand resting on top of the other. Breathe in looking forward, then breathe out and gently twist toward the left. Breathe in and return forward, then breathe out and twist right.

Repetitions: 3 on each side

Lazy Stretch

Gently stretches backs of legs; limbers lower back and neck

Bend your knees and rest your forearms on your knees, hands clasped. Breathe in and look up,

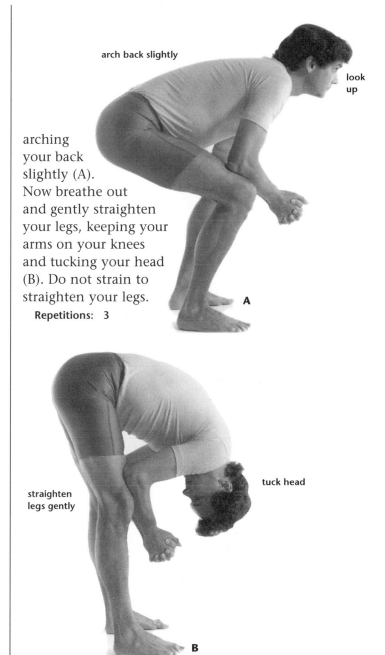

arching your back slightly (A). Now breathe out and gently straighten your legs, keeping your arms on your knees and tucking your head (B). Do not strain to straighten your legs.

Repetitions: 3

Standing Reach (pictured, p. 84, top left)

Breathe out completely, arms at your sides. Breathe in and reach over your head, stretch up, then breathe out and lower arms.

Repetitions: 3

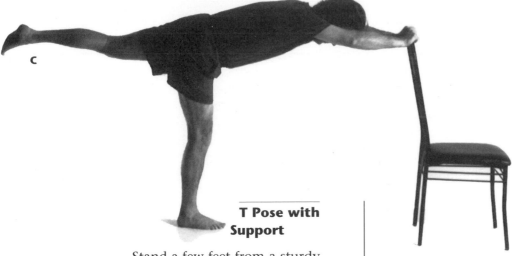

T Pose with Support

Stand a few feet from a sturdy chair or counter. Reach forward, bending your torso parallel to the floor and holding on to the chair with both hands. Breathe in and slowly lift your left leg to the back, parallel to the floor, or as high as you can (C). Hold for a few seconds, then breathe out and lower the leg. Repeat with the right leg.

Repetitions: **3 on each side.**

Baby Pose *(pictured, p. 46)*

Kneel on the floor, sitting back on your heels, and slowly lower your head to the floor. Let your arms rest at your sides with the elbows bent outward. Settle into the most comfortable position. Relax completely for at least 1 minute. If this pose is not comfortable due to stiff hips or knees, try one of the variations on page 81 or rest lying on your back, in the Corpse Pose.

Cat Breath *(pictured, p. 74)*

On hands and knees, breathe in as you arch your back and look up. Breathe out as you round your back and tuck your head.

Repetitions: **3**

Arm and Leg Balance

Strengthens muscles of the lower and midback; strengthens legs and hips

On hands and knees, breathe out completely. Then breathe in and raise your left arm and right leg parallel to the floor (D). Look straight ahead at your

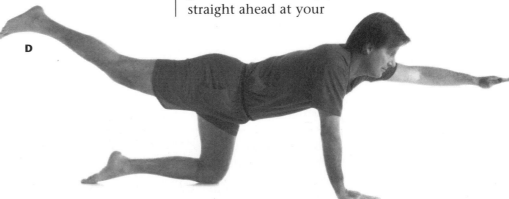

outstretched arm or, if your balance is shaky, stare at one spot on the floor. Breathe out and lower arm and leg. Repeat with the right arm and left leg.

Repetitions: 3 on each side

Knee Squeeze—Single *(pictured, p. 86)*

Lie on your back with arms overhead. Breathe in and raise your left knee, grasp it with both hands, lift your head, and hold your breath in as you squeeze the knee to your chest. Breathe out and relax back to your starting position.

Repetitions: 3 on each side

Knee Squeeze—Double

If you have lower back problems, begin this exercise with knees bent and feet on the floor. Breathe in and lift both knees to your chest, grasp them with both hands, lift your head, and hold your breath in as you squeeze the knees to your chest. Breathe out and lower to your starting position.

Repetitions: 3

Floor Stretch *(pictured, p. 111)*

Lie on your back with arms over your head. Gently stretch your left arm upward and your left leg downward, keeping feet flexed and pushing your heels away from you. Repeat with the right arm and leg. Then stretch both arms and legs. Do not strain.

Repetitions: once on each side, once on both sides

Easy Bridge *(pictured, p. 49)*

Lie on your back with knees bent and feet several inches apart. Your arms should be at your sides, palms down. Breathe out completely, pushing your waist to the floor slightly, then breathe in and lift your hips, arching your back. Be sure to keep your neck and shoulders relaxed. Do not strain. Breathe out and lower.

Repetitions: 3

Easy Cobra

Gently limbers entire spine; balances both halves of body; improves circulation; massages all internal organs

Lie on your stomach, resting on your forearms with hands clasped and elbows on the floor just below your shoulders, fairly close to your body. Breathe out and let your head and upper back relax forward (E). Now breathe in and lift your head and eyes up and back as far as possible without strain, then continue breathing in, arching your back and stretching up on your elbows, so you feel a slight

let shoulders, neck, and head relax

E

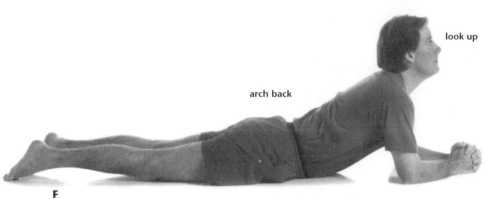

look up

arch back

F

stomach stays on floor

stretch along your entire spinal column (F). Do not strain. Breathe out and relax your back, then your head and eyes. Caution: This exercise should not be done if you have had recent surgery, have an open cut anywhere on your body, or by women during the menstrual cycle.

Repetitions: 3

Alternate Back Strengthener

Strengthens back and hips; massages internal organs

Lie on your stomach with arms stretched overhead and your forehead on the floor. Breathe out. Breathe in as you raise your left arm, right leg, and head (G). Breathe out and lower.

Repetitions: 3 on each side

Boat Pose *(pictured, p. 95)*

Lie on your stomach with arms overhead and forehead on the floor. Breathe out completely. Breathe in and lift arms, legs, and head, looking up. Breathe out and lower.

Repetitions: 3

G

RELAXATION AND MEDITATION: 8 MINUTES

The best meditation position for back and neck problems is lying flat with pillows under your thighs to release pressure on your lower back. Do not put a pillow under your head or neck. If the hardness of the floor is uncomfortable, lie on a foam mat.

Age or Convalescence

If you've been bedridden for some time, or if you're an older person and haven't exercised in a while, you can still practice Yoga very profitably and enjoyably. The following routine will help you gradually get into the habit of exercising. Even if you're bedridden, you can do the breathing techniques and the relaxation and meditation. And if you can wiggle your toes, you can do Yoga!

This workout starts in bed. If you're recovering, sometimes it takes a while to get up. Your muscles are stiff, or weak from not being used much. The exercises will help to prevent bedsores by increasing circulation. Circulation also brings fresh blood to your brain and can change your mood. It's easy to get depressed when you're ill or infirm; the days are long, and there are few diversions. Yoga techniques can lift depression and boredom. This workout can be done more than once a day.

The routine graduates to sitting up on the side of your bed, and finally, if you're able, to a few standing positions. Meditation can be done either lying in bed or sitting in a chair that supports your back while keeping it straight.

IN BED

Complete Breath (full description, pp. 28–29)

Lie flat, without pillows under your head if possible. You may bend your knees, separate your feet slightly, and let your knees touch. Breathe in and out evenly and smoothly, concentrating on the sound of the breath. Keep breathing for about 2 minutes.

Repetitions: **5-10**

Knee Squeeze (pictured, p. 86)

If you don't have room to stretch your arms overhead, leave them at your sides. Breathe out first, then breathe in, lift your head, and lift one leg toward your chest. Grasp the knee with both hands and hold your breath in as you squeeze the knee to your chest. Breathe out and lower the leg.

Repetitions: **3 on each side**

Ankle Rotations and Point-Flexes (pictured, p. 106)

Rotate your ankles several times in each direction. Point and flex your feet several times.

Repetitions: **5-6 circles in each direction, 5-6 point-flexes**

Knee Swings (pictured, p. 77)

Lying on your back, bend your knees and separate your feet. Bend both knees toward the left, then swing them over toward the right, gently stretching your lower back, stomach, and hips. Move slowly and carefully.

Repetitions: **5-10 on each side**

SITTING ON THE EDGE OF THE BED OR IN A CHAIR

Arched Breath (pictured, p. 27)

Rest your hands on your knees. Breathe in and arch your back, looking up and leaning forward slightly. Breathe out and round your back, tucking your head.

Repetitions: 3

Shoulder Roll *(pictured, p. 104)*

Let your arms hang loose at your sides. Rotate your shoulders several times in each direction.

Repetitions: 3-4 in each direction

Elbow Touch *(pictured, p. 104)*

With fingers touching your shoulders, breathe out and bring your elbows together in front, then breathe in and stretch your elbows toward the back.

Repetitions: 3

STANDING

Supported Leg Lift

Hold on to a sturdy chair or counter for support. Breathe out completely. Breathe in and lift your right leg straight ahead, keeping both knees straight (H).

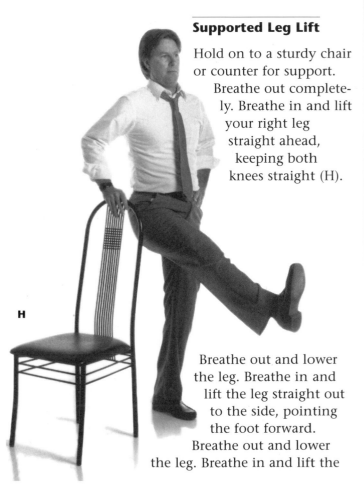

Breathe out and lower the leg. Breathe in and lift the leg straight out to the side, pointing the foot forward. Breathe out and lower the leg. Breathe in and lift the

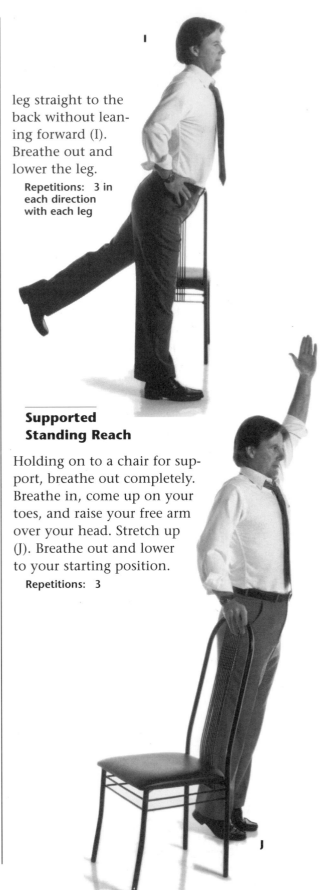

leg straight to the back without leaning forward (I). Breathe out and lower the leg.

Repetitions: 3 in each direction with each leg

Supported Standing Reach

Holding on to a chair for support, breathe out completely. Breathe in, come up on your toes, and raise your free arm over your head. Stretch up (J). Breathe out and lower to your starting position.

Repetitions: 3

RELAXATION AND MEDITATION

Meditate lying on a firm bed or sitting in a chair with back support. If you are lying down, do not put a pillow under your head. You can put a few pillows under your thighs to relieve pressure on your lower back.

Joint Disease or Injury

Most authorities recommend that arthritis sufferers engage in some form of exercise to keep the joints as limber as possible. Yoga is ideal because it is a gentle stretch that does not aggravate the condition. Yoga exercises improve circulation so that the muscles and joints get more nutrients, and toxins such as lactic acid are flushed out. Yoga exercise maintains muscle tone and range of motion of the joints. Breathing and meditation techniques teach you how to relax your muscles at will and how to reduce stress reactions that can aggravate already strained muscles.

A rule of thumb for joint pain is to exercise gently except when the joint is severely inflamed, such as during a severe attack of rheumatoid arthritis. Some pain may be experienced, but you can usually differentiate between extreme pain that is injuring the joint further and the aches of normal movement due to the swelling or stiffness of the joint. Pay particular attention to how your body feels during the exercise. Massage the joints thoroughly. Since a muscle strain usually is not felt until some time later—even as long as two days later in some cases—start with performing each exercise at about half capacity. The important thing is to keep moving, not to stretch as far as you can or strain to look like the picture in the book. Put the extra time into breathing and meditation.

With a few variations, you will be able to do the regular 20-minute workout. Your breathing segment will be the same. In the warm-up segment, if you have shoulder inflammation or injury, eliminate the Full Bend Variation and do the Shoulder Roll and Arm Roll very slowly, using small motions. In the exercise segment, if you have a hip injury, substitute a gentle Hip Rock and Rotation (see page 85) for the Twisting Triangle, eliminate the Tortoise Stretch, and substitute

the Knee Squeeze (page 86) for the Alternate Toe Touch. If you have inflammation or injury in the knee joint, grasp the thigh in the Knee Squeeze instead of the knee (K).

MASSAGE

The warmth and friction of massage help to bring blood into the joints and muscles while relaxing the muscles and connective tissue. If you have regular access to a massage therapist, take advantage of it. But if not, you can massage many of your own joints (L). Don't worry about exerting pressure;

the point is to warm the joint. Use your whole hand, not just your fingers, and rub the joint all over with slow, rhythmic, circular motions until you feel the skin warming. Massage each joint for at least a minute.

High Blood Pressure and Heart Disease

Yoga is gaining increasing recognition for its effectiveness in preventing and even, in some cases, reversing heart disease. One insurance company now reimburses patients for participation in a heart disease treatment program involving Yoga exercise and meditation, and others will no doubt follow suit.

Depending on the severity of your condition, you may be able to do the full regular workout. If your doctor says you shouldn't do forward-bending exercises, substitute the Standing Twist (page 105) for the Standing Sun Pose, do the Baby Pose supported on pillows (see page 81) and substitute the Knee Squeeze (see page 86) for the Easy Bridge. This routine will improve circulation and elasticity of the blood vessels. Breathing and meditation will be your best tools, because they teach you how to reduce stress reactions, relax at will, and keep your awareness on the present moment.

Chronic Fatigue Syndrome (CFS)

Unlike many exercise programs, Yoga practice does not take energy away from the system; instead, it puts energy back into the system. Whereas many exercise programs leave you exhausted, your Yoga exercise period will leave you refreshed and renewed. Yoga exercises combined with breathing and meditation techniques provide a daily support system that makes a normal, productive life possible for those with CFS. I recall one young woman who was ready to quit her job with a brokerage house due to CFS; she found that practicing Yoga every morning gave her the energy to keep up with the demands of a regular work schedule.

Here's how it works: Physical and emotional tension and fatigue lodge in muscle tissue, making it knotted and hot, and the circulation sluggish. Yoga exercises systematically stretch and relax the major muscle groups and push fresh blood and oxygen through the tissues, which releases the tension and allows the muscles to relax and cool. The exercises are done slowly, and the breathing patterns with each exercise allow for maximum oxygen intake and for the release of toxins.

Breathing techniques improve concentration and awareness, and help to reduce stress reactions that are expressed in the body. Extreme reactions to stress cause energy demands to increase rapidly. Your breathing techniques put you in touch with the untapped strength and energy that lie within you. By constantly returning the mind to the present moment in meditation, you allow the body to deal with what's happening now.

Relaxation and meditation teach conservation of energy and build self-confidence. You learn to completely relax every muscle in your body and then to forget about the body while turning attention toward the mind in meditation.

In meditation you simply stop all thought momentarily, allowing your inner strength to express itself.

If you have chronic fatigue syndrome, daily practice of the regular 20-minute workout (or any of the variations in this book), preferably in the morning, will give you the energy you need to be happy and creative.

Asthma

There are many theories about what causes the frightening tightness in the chest, the wheezing, and the difficulty breathing that characterize asthma attacks. Some authorities blame stress; others cite pollution or sensitivity to allergens. But whatever the cause, more and more sufferers from asthma are turning to Yoga for relief. Yoga breathing exercises, especially, help reduce the symptoms of asthma in several ways.

By strengthening and relaxing the muscles of the lungs, the nerve activity in the airways is reduced, causing less constriction during an asthma attack. Also, through daily practice of rhythmic, controlled breathing techniques, the respiratory muscles and lungs develop the ability to breathe more slowly all the time, resulting in less stress on the airways in general.

Regular practice of the complete relaxation technique (see Chapter 5) allows you to be more aware of when and where your body holds tension so that you can consciously relax it. Developing a more relaxed physical body seems to reduce the incidence and severity of asthma attacks.

The following 20-minute workout concentrates on exercises that stretch and relax the respiratory muscles while using several specific breathing patterns to control and relax the breath. Practice it every day if you are affected by attacks often. As your attacks decrease, you should be able to practice the regular workout most days, and do the special asthma routine once or twice a week.

When you feel an attack coming on, the first thing to do is relax completely. Check the places in your body that hold tension the most—probably your face, shoulders, and stomach. Consciously relax. Then sit straight—on the edge of a chair is fine—and do a few concentrated Complete Breaths. As you breathe, don't think about anything except the sound of the breath and the feeling of the breath moving in and out slowly, deeply, and rhythmically.

In your breathing segment, after the Arched Breath, add the following two exercises designed to stretch the respiratory muscles and improve the length and smoothness of the Complete Breath:

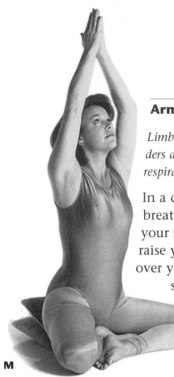

M

Arm Reach

Limbers and releases tension in shoulders and upper back; improves respiration

In a comfortable seated position, breathe out with your arms at your sides, then breathe in and raise your arms in a wide circle over your head. Look up and stretch (M). Breathe out and lower your arms.

Repetitions: 3 or more

Arm Swing

Limbers and releases tension in upper back; improves respiration

In a comfortable seated position, stretch arms straight in front of you with palms together (N). Breathe out. Breathe in as you stretch your arms to the sides and back as far as possible without strain (O).

Repetitions: 3 or more

N

Dancer Pose *(pictured, p. 63)*

Stand next to a sturdy chair or a wall for support. Stare at one spot for balance. Grasp your right foot in your left hand, steady yourself, then carefully lift the right foot up and back, and raise your right arm straight up next to your ear. Relax your stomach and your breath. Hold for several seconds. Repeat on the other side.

Repetitions: 1 on each side

Stretching Dog

Limbers lower back and hips; stretches backs of legs; increases circulation to head

Sit on your heels, toes tucked under and hands on the floor a few inches in front of your knees. Breathe in and arch your back,

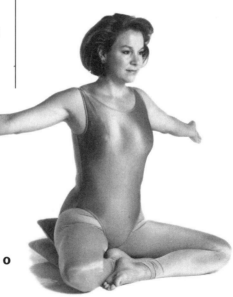

O

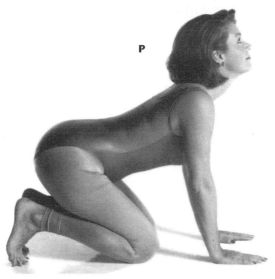

P

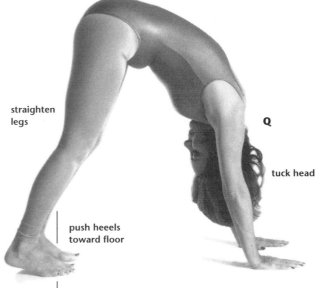

straighten
legs

Q

tuck head

push heeels
toward floor

looking up (P). Breathe out
and straighten your legs,
pushing your body into a V
position (Q). Tuck your
head.

Repetitions: 3

Diamond Pose *(pictured, p. 87)*

Sit straight with knees bent and
the soles of your feet touching.
Grasp your ankles with both
hands and rest your elbows on or
above your thighs. Breathe in
completely, then breathe out as
you lean forward slightly and press
down on your thighs with your
arms. Release.

Repetitions: 3

Now lace your fingers around your
toes, breathe in, and straighten
your spine. Breathe out as you
bend forward, letting your elbows
fall outside your legs this time.
Hold for a few seconds, then
breathe in and come back up.

Repetitions: 3

Seated Sun Pose *(pictured, p. 94)*

Sit straight with both legs
stretched in front, toes pulled back
toward your face, arms at your
sides. Breathe in as you lift your
arms to the sides and overhead.
Look up and stretch, elongating
your spine. Then breathe out and
bend forward over your legs, tucking your head. Grasp your ankles
with both hands (or, if you can
reach your toes comfortably, grasp
the toes as shown on page 48).
Bend your arms and pull gently.
Hold for a few seconds. Then
release, breathe in, and bring your
arms in another circle to the sides
and overhead. Look up. Breathe
out and lower your arms to your
sides.

Repetitions: 3

Extended Hero Pose

Stretches rib cage; improves respiration; limbers upper back and shoulders

In a kneeling position, clasp your hands behind you and straighten your arms (R). Breathe in completely. Breathe out and bend forward, keeping your arms straight and pulled away from your body as much as possible (S). Breathe in and come back up.

Repetitions: 3

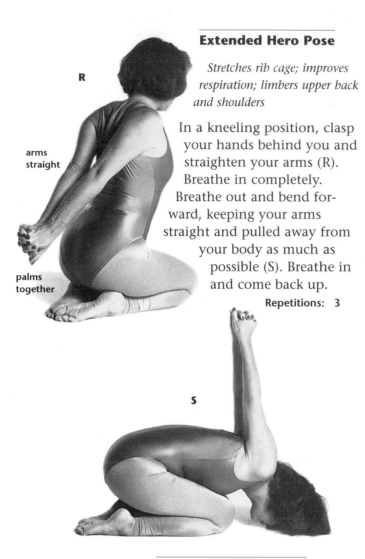

R

arms straight

palms together

S

Cat Breath *(pictured, p. 74)*

On hands and knees, breathe in as you arch your back and look up. Breathe out as you round your back and tuck your head.

Repetitions: 3

Camel Pose *(pictured, p. 110)*

Kneel with legs slightly separated. The first 2 movements help to prepare the spine for an intense stretch: Carefully bend back and grasp your left heel with your left hand. Push your hips forward slightly. Repeat on the right side. Now bend backward and grasp one heel with each hand. Push your

hips forward as far as possible and let your head relax back. Hold for several seconds, breathing normally. Release.

Repetitions: 1

Baby Pose *(pictured, p. 46)*

Easy Bridge *(pictured, p. 49)*

Lie on your back with knees bent and feet several inches apart. Place your hands, palms down, next to your body, or grasp your ankles. Relax your neck and shoulders, breathe in and lift your hips, arching your back. Hold a moment, then breathe out and lower.

Repetitions: 3

Knee Squeeze *(pictured, p. 86)*

Lie on your back with arms overhead. Breathe out, then breathe in and lift your head as you bring one leg toward your chest. Grasp the knee with both hands and hold your breath in as you squeeze the knee to your chest. Breathe out and lower the leg.

Repetitions: 3 on each side

Cobra Pose *(pictured, p. 46)*

Lie on your stomach with forehead on the floor and hands under your shoulders, palms down, elbows up. Breathe out completely. Breathe in and slowly curl up, starting with your head and eyes, then your chest, then your stomach. Use your back muscles; don't straighten your arms. Breathe out and curl down, starting with the stomach; keep your head and eyes back until the very last.

Repetitions: 3

Substance Abuse Recovery

Any kind of addiction can be helped by the discipline and health of regular Yoga practice. If you are trying to heal from an addiction, do everything you can to become healthy—starting with Yoga. Yoga will teach you techniques that you can use throughout the day to reinforce healthy habits. Most important, Yoga will shift your attention from the pain of withdrawal to the reassurance of knowing that you are on your way to recognizing the strength and power to change that is already a part of you. Addiction does not destroy your strength; it makes you forget about it. Yoga helps you remember and use it to grow healthy again.

Years ago, my teacher Rama was counseling one of my students who was trying to recover from a heroin addiction. He advised the student to practice the Archer Pose (page 65) every day and to chew on whole cloves all day. I have no scientific evidence to support this treatment, but I do know that it worked for that student and has worked for others since.

CAFFEINE

Caffeine is a potent drug. Besides its addictive properties, it is toxic to some people. The symptoms of caffeine toxicity resemble anxiety neurosis and may be misdiagnosed by unaware health care providers. Toxicity does not depend on ingesting large quantities of caffeine. Some people are sensitive to the relatively small amount of caffeine in just one cup of coffee or tea.

Because Yoga acts as a natural stimulant by increasing your energy level, you may find yourself cutting down on your caffeine intake without making a conscious decision to do so. As a general rule, you'll find that as you become stronger and healthier, your body will naturally tend to reject things that will harm it.

SLEEPING AIDS

Sleep-inducing drugs interfere with your body's natural sleep cycle and create a psychological dependence on the substance for going to sleep. If you have trouble falling asleep, practice your Complete Breath and the relaxation and meditation procedures while lying in bed. Many people have found this extremely helpful for getting back into a normal cycle of adequate rest at night. Often an inability to fall asleep simply means that you are unable to stop thinking about work; Yoga practice can teach you to stop working when you wish to.

Some people find their Yoga workout so energizing that they have trouble falling asleep if they practice in the evening. If you find that the exercise segment of the workout tends to wake you up, practice that portion of the routine in the morning instead, and continue doing the breathing and meditation just before going to sleep.

NICOTINE

If you're trying to stop smoking, the hardest part is finding a substitute for a cigarette when you feel

YOGA AND YOUR DIET

If you are trying to improve your health by practicing Yoga, it doesn't make sense to counteract these beneficial effects by feeding yourself junk.

There are many fine books that can give you detailed information about how to start eating better: I particularly recommend any book by Adelle Davis. Although her books were written mostly in the 1950s and 1960s, they were based on such solid research that they are still valuable today. I have never found her advice to be unhelpful. You may also benefit from consulting a nutritionist or practitioner of holistic medicine. Especially if you are attempting to switch to a vegetarian diet, it's important to make sure you are eating a balanced diet that includes enough protein. I do not recommend macrobiotic diets; many of my students who tried them developed nutritional deficiencies.

under stress. The Complete Breath is your best weapon against the urge to smoke. Simply start breathing deeply, using the three-stage procedure (see pages 28–29), and focus on the sound of the breath without thinking of anything else for a minute or so. The Complete Breath will relax you, temporarily take your mind off whatever is causing the stress reaction, and give you time to recover. You can do this breathing technique anywhere, anytime, and no one has to know you're doing it.

In addition to practicing the Complete Breath whenever you can, do your regular 20-minute workout daily to build up resistance to stress. As you learn new ways of coping, your craving for nicotine will diminish.

SUGAR

Although sugar is not truly chemically addictive, too much of it will cause your body to look for more as a substitute for what it really needs—energy to function. When you feel a craving for sugar, your body is asking for an energy boost. If you feed it sugar, you are giving it a quick fix, but you will pay the price in an energy letdown later. Instead, give your body extra protein and B vitamins, and practice your Yoga workout every day. You'll soon find yourself naturally reducing the amount of sweet things that you consume.

11

GETTING THE MOST FROM YOUR WORKOUT

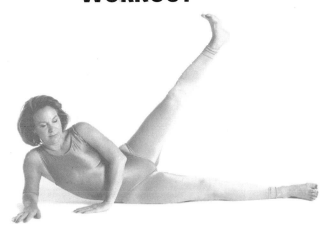

In Yoga, the push to health and well-being doesn't just click on at the beginning of your daily 20-minute workout and click off at the end. If you're like most people, you'll find that you want to tune up the rest of your life to harmonize with the benefits you're feeling from Yoga practice.

Yoga teaches you how to find your personal source of confidence and strength and how to activate these qualities. Join with that power source within you: practice your 20-minute workout daily, and follow the guidelines outlined in this chapter. You will find very quickly that your concentrated effort results in the ability to be the person you want to be, because you are putting your full strength behind what you want. The word Yoga means "union" in the Sanskrit language. When you practice Yoga, you are joining yourself to your power source within.

The first part of this chapter, "How to Make Each Day New," offers some helpful hints on how to keep your routine fresh and interesting so you can build up the self-discipline to practice happily every day. The second section, "10 Ways to Be Your Own Best Friend," is based on the ethical guidelines of Yoga. These are the building blocks to a strong and powerful personality that will work along with physical Yoga techniques to give you the power to become the person you want to be.

How to Make Each Day New

Concentration is naturally more intense while you are first learning a new thing, especially if it is something you have chosen to do. Many people feel elated and euphoric for the first weeks or months that they practice Yoga—because of the time, attention, and concentration they are putting in as well as because of the results they are feeling.

But at some point, the question comes up: *So what do I do next?* After you have learned the workout, the basic techniques essentially remain the same throughout practice. Of course there are different *asans* that can be learned over the course of many months of practice, and various breathing techniques, but eventually, every daily routine includes some breathing, warming up, a sequence of exercises, and a period of relaxation and meditation. Some people stop practicing when the newness has worn off because they don't feel as euphoric as in the beginning. When the most obvious results level off, they don't believe the techniques are working anymore. But Yoga has many subtle effects, very few of which are apparent at first to the conscious mind. As you continue practicing, you will begin to notice things that have changed in ways that were not so obvious at first. You may notice yourself standing straighter and moving more easily, for instance. You may notice yourself choosing healthier food to eat. You may notice yourself not reacting so sharply to upsets or anxieties. Most important, you may notice more willpower, creativity, attention to detail, and self-confidence.

The key to conquering boredom in Yoga practice is to develop the awareness and appreciation that make each technique feel new and special. Sometimes this takes imagination. After you have done the Standing Sun Pose a dozen times, you don't have to think about how to breathe, where to put your hands, how to hold your legs— your body does it automatically. So where does your mind go? Your shopping list, your kids, your job, whatever. The frenetic activity of the mind seems almost like a hamster running endlessly inside a wheel. Now is the time to trick your mind a bit. Use the principles of meditation: stop all thought while exercising. When you return to thought, it will be different.

It does no good to force yourself into a drudging sort of mind-set, where you do the routine each day because *you think you should*. That drags down the inspiration of Yoga and loads it with guilt. Guilt has no place in Yoga. Why do anything you don't enjoy? And if you *want* to enjoy something, there are ways to change your perception of that thing.

Here are some ideas for breathing new life into your daily practice:

Vary your 20-minute workout. This book contains many different 20-minute workout variations. Even though some of them may not apply to you (for instance, the workout to do while traveling), try them once in a while for a change of pace.

Face a different wall, or practice in a different room. How simple this is! It gives you a new perspective on everything, from the feel of a different carpet to a different point of view. Face out a window. You'll see, but not really see, the view, but this slight mental abstraction will help you slip into meditation much more easily.

Try a different time of day. Unless it's impossible because of work or family schedules, try shifting to evening if you've been practicing in the morning, or vice versa. You will find that your mind feels different, as does your body.

Do some exercises more slowly. Try the 8-count breath with some of the exercises and perform them as if you were under water or in a slow-motion film sequence.

Watch your breath. Concentrating on the sound of your breath works very quickly to focus your attention. Most people find that when they practice this way, their entire exercise routine becomes almost as still and focused as meditation.

Vary the order of the techniques. The workout is ordered in such a way as to gradually focus your mind toward meditation, which is last in the sequence. But this is not required. Rearrange the order of the techniques and see what you feel.

Keep a journal. Many people keep a record of their feelings, thoughts, dreams, and experiences when starting Yoga practice. This is very helpful for noticing many things, such as how the exercises are affecting your health, the length or smoothness of your breath, your experiences in meditation, and how the workout is affecting the rest of your day. I have had many students complain to me after several months that they have not made any progress. When I point out to them what I observe—that their skin is clearer, their walk is more graceful and relaxed, their life in better order than it was—they are amazed, because the changes happened so gradually they didn't notice. A journal is a way to notice these things yourself.

Write to me. I love hearing from students who are using my materials. If you tell me what you are doing, often I can suggest some way to give you an extra challenge or offer a new perspective on some problem or experience.

Stop practicing for a week. I'm serious! If you are not enjoying what you are doing, stop it cold. Don't do *anything* related to Yoga for a week—and be firm. Probably you will find that you miss it after a few days, but wait the full week. Think about what it is you miss, and how you feel each day. When you do go back to practicing daily, you'll enjoy it that much more.

10 Ways to Be Your Own Best Friend

Many people who begin practicing Yoga wonder about the philosophy that supports Yoga. I feel that it is not productive to dissociate theory from practice, so throughout this book, I have tried to introduce you to some of the most important concepts in Yoga as they relate to your experiences in your daily 20-minute Yoga workout. There is one very important aspect of Yoga philosophy, however, that merits a more lengthy discussion.

A line in *The Bhagavad Gita* (a short section from a very long Indian epic called *The Mahabharata*) tells us that we can be our own best friend or our own worst enemy. By our actions, reactions, and habits; how we handle stress; and how we view our successes and problems, we can either help our lives run more smoothly or fight ourselves all the way. One way to short-circuit resistance is through the practice of ethics. In Yoga, ethical behavior is the cornerstone of progress. Practicing ethics in Yoga is not done in order to produce a good, socially conscious individual, or in order to abide by an external moral code, but to reduce mental and emotional disturbances. Ethical behavior frees you to become productive and creative, to achieve optimum physical and mental health, and to move through the world with appreciation and grace—filled with the strength and power to be the person you want to be and do what you want to do. Yoga points out that you have a choice.

In Yoga, ethics includes 10 general guidelines. These are complex ideas, worth the time to study and put into practice. Studying and experimenting with these guidelines will give more depth and meaning to your 20-minute workout. Choose a different one each month, write it on a piece of paper and post it on your refrigerator, and check your attitudes and feelings each day. Following is a brief summary of the most relevant aspects of each guideline:

1 *Don't harm yourself or others (Nonviolence)*

This is first on the list because it is the most important. There are so many ways in which we harm ourselves either consciously or unconsciously: by driving with someone who has been drinking; by using drugs or smoking or using alcohol to excess; by not getting enough rest; by eating the wrong foods, or eating too much or not enough. Guard against these types of destructive activities that are motivated by self-hatred. Avoid any action or omission that interferes with your health and well-being. If one of your goals is improving your health by practicing Yoga, it makes sense to try to refrain from doing things that counteract that goal.

Don't harm yourself by causing harm to anyone else. Learn to be assertive rather than aggressive. Be aware of thoughts or actions of revenge—a subtle form of violence that does nobody any good. Violence hinders Yoga because it is based in fear, and fear prevents positive growth.

Many people misinterpret this ethic to mean that you must never get angry or upset if you practice Yoga. Impossible! Human beings will always have emotions, but when you practice nonviolence, your anger will not be destructive, and those to whom you are expressing your emotions will not be harmed. This ethic has the result of building an atmosphere of safety and confidence around you. When you've been consciously practicing nonviolence for a while, you will start to notice a greater feeling of peace, and it will affect those around you.

2 Don't lie to yourself and others (Truthfulness)

Telling the truth means, first and foremost, following through with what you say, even in casual conversation. Observe the promises you make to yourself—no matter how trivial—and how often you follow through. If you say to yourself, "I'll go to the grocery on my way home from work," do it. This is a way of becoming more conscious of what you think, say, and do. The awareness that you build by keeping your word will make your experience in meditation quieter and more focused. Serious Yoga practitioners are even careful of the jokes they make, because they know that concentrated thought and even speech can be very powerful. Because most people do not know themselves very well, they tend to believe what others tell them about themselves.

Over time, the practice of truthfulness reduces feelings of insecurity, self-hate, and fear, because when you tell the truth, you begin to know yourself better; you stop lying to yourself and accepting false views about yourself from others. Lying to yourself maintains a fantasy view of yourself that is not true. Being true to yourself means being yourself and enjoying the person you are.

One additional point needs to be made about truthfulness: Nonviolence always takes precedence. If telling the truth would harm someone, it is better to keep silent. My teacher, the great Lakshmanjoo of Kashmir, told me a story about a Yogi who lived in a forest and practiced these ethical guidelines fervently. One day a deer bounded in fright through the clearing where the Yogi lived. A few minutes later, a hunter came riding by. When he saw the Yogi, he stopped and asked, "Did you see a deer come by? Which way did it go?" The Yogi, bound by truth and nonviolence, answered, "The eyes have seen, but the eyes cannot speak. The mouth can speak, but the mouth cannot see."

3 Don't steal from yourself or others (Nonstealing)

Stealing happens only when, for some reason or another, we don't believe that we have enough—enough time, enough power, enough stuff. The urge to take, to possess, to own has to do with feeling separate. When you feel connected, you won't feel the desire for something that belongs to someone else, because your whole attitude of ownership will change. When you understand that everything you "own" is really a gift, lent to you for a time, you'll feel much more appreciative and less likely to feel lacking.

More important than stealing from others, however, is the tendency to steal from yourself. Unawareness, which Lakshmanjoo has called "the thief of the mind," steals the experience of the present moment. Wasting time steals the opportunity to learn something. Self-destructive behavior steals your health and happiness.

4 Be respectful and aware of sexual desire in yourself (Avoiding promiscuity)

Be aware of how important love is to you. One of the important concepts in Yoga is becoming aware of what thoughts, feelings, and memories occupy your mind, so that you can choose what to think about. In this way your willpower is strengthened and you have more energy to do or think about the things that are most important in your life, instead of your attention being frittered away on unproductive thought. Thus the Yoga practitioner learns to focus thought in fewer directions; the mind becomes less scattered.

One of the most frequent thoughts and feelings to go through everyone's mind has to do with sex. It is so prevalent that you probably don't even realize it is there most of the time. Sexual thought is enhanced, stimulated, and prodded by the media. Every television commercial that features a beautiful woman or man is using the power of sex to associate the product with exciting feelings. In Yoga, sometimes the temporary practice of celibacy is suggested in order to help students become more aware of their thoughts and desires. You can try this yourself by taking a 5-minute "celibacy break" at some time every day. During those 5 minutes, observe every thought and feeling that goes through your mind, especially when you are interacting with another person, and see if you can pull back from sexual associations just for that 5-minute period.

Please understand that this ethic does not intend to take sex away from your life or convince you that it is bad or undesirable. Nothing could be further from the truth! In Yoga, especially the Shaivistic philosophy taught to me by Lakshmanjoo, the world in all its complexity is embraced, not discarded. Far from making sex less desirable to you, you will probably find that this regular celibacy break improves your enjoyment of sex because of your greater awareness. A small amount of celibacy practice gives you great appreciation for both sex and love.

Celibacy is also practiced sometimes in order to allow one person's personality to become strong enough not to be absorbed into another's. This often happens in a love relationship; people become so attached to and identify so strongly with their partner that they lose their own identity. After a divorce, a short period of celibacy can help heal a person by restoring the sense of self-worth that has been damaged by the feelings of rejection and acrimony resulting from a breakup.

5 *Simplify the things you want and need (Nonpossessiveness)*

This ethic is not about giving away all your possessions! In Yoga, it's not what you have but how you feel about it that matters. It takes a balanced outlook: in the ideal state of mind, you would be responsible and careful with your possessions, invest your money wisely, and so on, but you would also think more clearly about what you value and why. Practicing this ethic will show you where you put your time and energy and where your priorities lie.

This ethic also applies to our desire to see results from our actions. All of us have goals when we practice Yoga, and it is natural to want results. But in Yoga, paradoxically, the way to get results is *not to look for results constantly*. Do all the preparatory work—the exercises, breathing, meditation, following these ethics—but without demanding a particular result. This opens up at least two wonderful possibilities for you. First, by not limiting yourself to a particular goal, you allow the opportunity for something even better to occur. Important values emerge that you may not have realized before. Second, your practice becomes less frantic, because you are enjoying the practice itself instead of running after some imagined future result like the donkey running after the carrot. It's like putting your car on cruise control and then enjoying the ride.

6 Make yourself as clear and healthy as possible (Purity)

Forget the religiously toned injunctions about absolute cleanliness of body and mind that you may have heard. There is no need at this time to do elaborate "cleansing" rituals in order to practice Yoga with this book. Use your ethics concerning purity to make yourself as healthy, strong, beautiful, and disciplined as you can. Make your surroundings clean, pleasant, and orderly. Eat foods that contribute to health and well-being. Balance work and play in your life. Be disciplined about daily practice. Invest in some counseling or therapy to understand yourself better and to help you gain new tools to deal with the psychological blocks to your well-being.

7 Practice being happy with who you are and what you are (Contentment)

In meditation, as you have learned, focusing on the present moment is the way to achieve the best state of relaxation and quietness. You can also practice this awareness and enjoyment of the present moment in every aspect of life. When you observe the

thoughts and feelings and desires that flood your mind every day, you'll notice that many have to do with either the past or the future. If you can practice constantly bringing your mind back to the present, you'll enjoy life a lot more—not only will it seem to slow down, but because your attention is on what's happening right now instead of what might or could be or has been or would have been in the past or future, you'll notice more about yourself and others and enjoy the experience of each day. More important, freeing yourself from anxiety about past and future will eliminate a great many of your stress reactions.

Contentment also has to do with feeling connected to yourself and the world around you—but it is not dependent on anything outside of you; it cannot exist with separateness. Contentment does not include any conditions ("I'd be happy if only I had . . . "), but it is not the same as not wanting anything. You may want good health, for example, but the true feeling of contentment does not depend on your being healthy. Contentment is learning to be happy with who you are and what you are right now.

At the same time, this ethic does not mean that you do not change; on the contrary, change is a permanent part of life and especially of Yoga practice. Change forces you to grow, and you gain a greater tolerance of the way things are. Yoga helps you discover freedom and the power to change. Learn what gives you happiness; make positive changes in that direction, and then learn to be happy as you change.

Once, in Kashmir, I was sympathizing with Lakshmanjoo when he told me he had to have some dental work done. He smiled and said, "I have two choices. I can hate it or I can enjoy it. I choose to enjoy!"

8 Learn more about what's important to you (Study)

No one practices best in a vacuum. If you're intrigued with some of the ideas you've read about in this book, take it one step further: read some of the books mentioned in the Appendix and learn more about how Yoga works and some of the philosophy behind Yoga practice. Study increases your substance and broadens your capacity for experience. Study every day, for a few minutes at least, so that you can be confident that you're increasing your depth of self-knowledge.

9 Encourage heroic capability in yourself (Tolerance)

All over the world, mythological systems celebrate the hero who sets out on seemingly impossible adventures and returns with capacities or ideas that benefit the entire community. The definition of a hero is one who keeps on taking just one more step. A hero has the courage to keep on trying in the face of formidable obstacles.

In Yoga, you are the hero, and the trials and adventures that you face are the processes of learning self-discipline, continuity, applying the techniques where they are needed, and improving your powers of concentration. By practicing Yoga, for example, you learn not to give in to the ravages of stress; instead, you learn techniques to reduce the effects of the stress

reactions you experience. In mythological terms, you "conquer" the "dragon" of uncontrolled stress reactions with your "sword" of breathing, exercise, and relaxation techniques that reduce those reactions.

The hero recognizes that as one mission is accomplished, there is always another, and the way to succeed is to keep taking one step at a time. By the same token, the hero recognizes that failure is inevitable on the road to success, and the true hero learns to fail with poise. Many people fear failure mostly because they do not want to look bad. The hero realizes that one can fail and still look good; the failure—even if it is a big failure—does not take anything away from the fact of taking one more step; of being true to oneself; of looking forward, not back; of believing in yourself.

This attitude builds strength and stamina, physically and mentally. You can always do a little more than you think you can. When you are able to do this, make a note of your achievement and appreciate yourself and your efforts.

10 See yourself in a larger picture (Remembrance)

It may seem odd that "remembrance" is in this list of ethics. What does remembrance have to do with behavior? Practicing remembrance means seeing yourself as part of a much bigger picture and respecting your place in that pattern. When you consider the enormity of the universe, you may feel small or insignificant, but that is a limited outlook that assumes you are separate. You are not separate. You are a vital part of this drama of life; whatever role you play, make it as happy and as perfect as you can. Don't look back on your life with guilt. Appreciate the diversity of the world. Try to respect all the qualities of life equally—good and bad, sweet and painful, beautiful and ugly, happy and sad. Learn to appreciate your life with sensitivity and awareness.

As you practice your 20-minute Yoga workout, enjoy the wonderful changes and opportunities that Yoga makes possible in your life. Enjoy the person you are and the person you are becoming. You are giving yourself a daily gift of health, well-being, and new awareness of the depth and capability of your self.

APPENDIX

RESOURCES FROM THE AMERICAN YOGA ASSOCIATION

Some instructional materials that you might find helpful for supplementing your 20-minute workout are available from the American Yoga Association. We would also be happy to send a teacher or lecturer to your area for a special program. Please write or call either of our two centers for more information.

For classes and programs in the Sarasota, Florida, area or for information about instructional materials:

AMERICAN YOGA ASSOCIATION
513 South Orange Avenue
Sarasota, Florida 34236
(813) 953-5859 (800) 226-5859

For classes and programs in the greater Cleveland area:

AMERICAN YOGA ASSOCIATION
P.O. Box 18105
Cleveland Heights, Ohio 44118
(216) 371-0078

Books and Tapes

BOOKS

The American Yoga Association Beginner's Manual. Complete instructions for over 90 Yoga exercises and breathing techniques; three 10-week curriculum outlines; and chapters on nutrition, philosophy, stress management, and more.

Conversations with Swami Lakshmanjoo, Volume I: *Aspects of Kashmir Shaivism.* Edited transcripts of Alice Christensen's interviews with Swami Lakshmanjoo, talking about his childhood and early years in Yoga, plus some basic concepts in the philosophy of Kashmir Shaivism.

Conversations with Swami Lakshmanjoo, Volume II: *The Yamas and Niyamas of Patanjali.* Edited transcripts of Alice Christensen's dialogues with Swami Lakshmanjoo about these essential ethical guidelines in Yoga.

Easy Does It Yoga. For those with physical limitations, this book includes instruction in specially adapted Yoga exercises that can be done in a chair or in bed, breathing techniques, and meditation.

Easy Does It Yoga Trainer's Guide. A complete manual for how to begin teaching the Easy Does It Yoga program to adults with physical limitations due to age, convalescence, substance abuse, injury, or obesity. Intended for health professionals, activities directors, physical therapists, home health aides, and others who work with the elderly or in rehabilitative services.

The Joy of Celibacy. This booklet examines how the unconscious is influenced by the sexual sell of modern advertising and suggests a 5-minute celibacy break to help build awareness and self-knowledge.

The Light of Yoga. A chronicle of the unusual circumstances that catapulted Alice Christensen into Yoga practice in the early 1950s, including the teachers and experiences that shaped her first years of study.

Meditation. A collection of excerpts from lectures and classes on the subject of meditation, including a section of questions and answers from students.

Reflections of Love. A collection of excerpts from Alice Christensen's lectures and classes on the subject of love.

AUDIOTAPES

Complete Relaxation and Meditation with Alice Christensen. A two-tape audiocassette program that features three guided meditation sessions of varying lengths, including instruction in a seated posture, plus a discussion of meditation experiences.

Songs of Bliss. Swami Rama sings traditional Sanskrit songs and mantrams.

VIDEOTAPES

Basic Yoga. A complete introduction to Yoga that includes exercise, breathing, and relaxation and meditation techniques. Provides detailed instruction in all the techniques, including variations for more or less flexibility. Features a 30-minute practice session in a Yoga class setting for a convenient routine to do daily.

Conversations with Swami Lakshmanjoo. A set of three videotapes in which Alice Christensen introduces Swami Lakshmanjoo and talks with him about his background, the philosophy of Kashmir Shaivism, and other topics in Yoga. (Some material corresponds to the book *Aspects of Kashmir Shaivism,* described above.)

"It's Never Too Late!" A 30-minute documentary about the Easy Does It Yoga program. Features experts on aging, including the late Maggie Kuhn of the Gray Panthers, then-Senator Lawton Chiles, and Dr. Robert Butler of the National Institutes of Health. Narrated by Mason Adams.

About the American Yoga Association

The American Yoga Association teaches a comprehensive and balanced program of Yoga that includes Hatha Yoga exercises and breathing techniques as well as meditation. Rather than stressing physical culture for its own sake, our core curriculum acknowledges the deeper possibilities of Yoga by teaching meditation and by encouraging the inner-directed awareness that eventually leads to greater self-knowledge. This reliance on individual experience and feeling is a central theme in the science of Yoga, and it underlies the philosophical system of Kashmir Shaivism that supports our line of teaching.

Our goal is to offer the highest-quality Yoga instruction possible. In addition to regularly scheduled classes and seminars, we offer instructional books and tapes.

INDEX

The first presentation of each exercise is in **boldface.**

ABOUT THE AUTHOR

*Alice Christensen stands out as a Yoga teacher
with the rare ability to make the often complex ideas
and techniques of Yoga accessible to our Western outlook and lifestyle. She established the American Yoga
Association in 1968, then the first and only
nonprofit educational organization teaching Yoga
in the United States.*

*For over 40 years, she has consistently
presented Yoga in a clear, classical manner, without
dogma or prescription, as a potent avenue for individual inquiry. She has designed programs of Yoga that
can be used to enhance any lifestyle. Whether the goal
is to maintain health or to explore the nature of the
self, her programs can be used to achieve a
wide range of goals.*